Rapid Revision in Endocrinology

Ben Greenstein
PhD MRPharmS BA(Hons) FRIH
Honorary Senior Research Fellow
Pain Management Service
Royal Free Hospital, London

Radcliffe Publishing
Oxford • New York

Radcliffe Publishing Ltd
18 Marcham Road
Abingdon
Oxon OX14 1AA
United Kingdom

www.radcliffe-oxford.com

Electronic catalogue and worldwide online ordering facility.

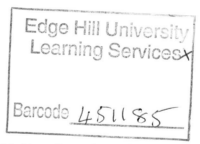
New research and clinical experience can result in changes in treatment
and drug therapy. Readers of this book should therefore check the most
recent product information on any drug they may prescribe to ensure they
are complying with the manufacturer's recommendations concerning
dosage, the method and duration of administration, and contraindications.
Neither the publisher nor the authors accept liability for any injury or
damage arising from this publication.

British Library Cataloguing in Publication Data

A catalogue record for this book is available from the British Library.

ISBN-13: 978 1 85775 794 1

Typeset by Anne Joshua & Associates, Oxford
Printed and bound by TJI Digital, Padstow, Cornwall

Contents

About the author

Ben Greenstein originally graduated as a Pharmacist in South Africa in 1965 and immigrated to the UK with his wife in 1966 where, after three years as a Community Pharmacist in London he obtained a PhD in Pharmacology at Chelsea College, University of London in 1975, studying molecular aspects of steroid hormone action. After carrying out endocrine research at Oxford University for three years as a Senior Research Fellow of the Mental Health Foundation, he took a post as lecturer in the Department of Pharmacology in St Thomas' Hospital Medical School (now absorbed into King's College, London) until 1992, after which he directed an endocrine research group studying endocrine aspects of lupus in the Lupus Research Unit in St Thomas' Hospital. In 1999 he moved to the Arizona Arthritis Center in the University of Arizona in Tucson as a Senior Visiting Research Professor, and returned to the UK in 2001, where he is currently a Visiting Senior Research Fellow in the Department of Pain Management Services. The author has produced text-books of pharmacology, endocrinology and neuroscience for undergraduate students, who are really the people who taught him everything he knows about those subjects.

Abbreviations

ACE	angiotensin-converting enzyme
Ach	acetylcholine
ACTH	adrenocorticotrophic hormone/corticotrophin
ADH	antidiuretic hormone, vasopressin
AMH	anti-Müllerian hormone
AVP	arginine vasopressin
BMD	bone mineral density
BMI	body mass index
BNF	*British National Formulary*
BPH	benign prostatic hyperplasia
CAH	congenital adrenal hyperplasia
CBG	corticosterone-binding globulin
CCK	cholecystokinin
CG	chorionic gonadotrophin
CNS	central nervous system
COCP	combined oral contraceptive pill
CRH	corticotrophin-releasing hormone
CSF	colony-stimulating growth factor
CT	computed tomography
DEXA	dual energy X-ray absorptiometry
DHEA	dehydroepiandrosterone
DHEAS	dehydroepiandrosterone sulphate
DHT	5α-dihydrotesosterone
DOC	deoxycorticosterone
DUBA	dual action bone agent
EGF	epidermal growth factor
FSH	follicle-stimulating hormone
GH	growth hormone
GHRH	growth-hormone-releasing hormone
GIT	gastrointestinal tract
GnRH	gonadotrophin-releasing hormone
GP	general practitioner
GRPP	glicentin-related polypeptide fragment
HCG	human chorionic gonadotrophin
HCS	chorionic somatomammotrophin (HPL)
HDL	high-density lipoprotein

HPL	human placental lactogen
HRT	hormone replacement therapy
IDDM	insulin-dependent diabetes mellitus
IGF	insulin-like growth factor
IGFBP	IGF-binding protein
IL-1	interleukin-1
IM	intramuscular
INF	interferon
IP_3	inositol triphosphate
IUD	intrauterine device
IV	intravenous
LATS	long-acting thyroid stimulator
LDL	low-density lipoprotein
LH	luteinising hormone
MEA	multiple endocrine adenomatosis
MEN	multiple endocrine neoplasia
MHC	major histocompatibility complex
MRI	magnetic resonance imaging
α-MSH	α-melanocyte-stimulating hormone
NGF	nerve growth factor
NIDDM	non-insulin-dependent diabetes mellitus
NK	natural killer
NSAID	non-steroidal anti-inflammatory drug
PAI	plasminogen activator inhibitor/primary adrenal insufficiency
PCOS	polycystic ovary syndrome
PDGF	platelet-derived growth factor
PIF	prolactin-inhibitory factor
PL	placental lactogen
PMS	premenstrual syndrome
PMT	premenstrual tension
POP	progestogen-only pill
PRL	prolactin
PTH	parathyroid hormone
PZI	protamin zinc insulin
RAA	renin angiotensin–aldosterone system
SERM	selective estrogen receptor modulator
SHBG	sex hormone-binding globulin
SLE	systemic lupus erythematosus
StAR	steroidogenic acute regulatory protein
STI	sexually transmitted infection
T_3	tri-iodothyronine
T_4	thyroxine

TBG	thyroxine-binding globulin
TBPA	thyroxine-binding pre-albumin
TGF	transforming growth factor
TH	thymocyte helper
TPR	total peripheral resistance
TRH	thyrotrophin-releasing hormone
TSH	thyroid-stimulating hormone/thyrotrophin
VIP	vasoactive intestinal peptide
VTE	venous thromboembolism
WHO	World Health Organization

For Lorraine

1 Introduction

This book is intended for the student in a hurry. It has been written by one who has experienced the terrors associated with the realisation that the examination is just around the corner. The writer is only too aware of the serious distractions and social pressures that conspire to keep students away from their books, and of the despair associated with the contemplation one week before an examination of a pile of unexplored and all too often hastily written lecture notes whose decipherment, let alone assimilation and digestion, presents a daunting challenge. The book also addresses the needs of the student who:

- at the beginning of an academic year needs a clear picture of the overall shape and size of the topic
- asks its relevance to the ultimate aim of the field of study
- may need direction as to how the information may be concisely and accessibly arranged in preparation for the day when it is called upon for examination purposes.

The reader will find here practical suggestions for the preparation of easily accessible notes which, from personal experience, the writer has found to be useful, particularly when *that* time of year comes around. These suggestions are offered in the knowledge that some readers prefer a more cursive style of information storage and retrieval, but it is hoped that some may find the method presented here useful.

Approaching the task in hand

Below are listed some of the printable exhortations used by this writer in order to help him get down to his revision (and writing this book):

- no one made me get into this
- I'm hoping this will help others
- it's better late than never
- at least I've got this book
- just think of that pass list
- I'm as good as the others
- this won't beat me
- either life's got its foot on my neck or I've got my foot on life's neck
- no one's going to do this for me.

Making notes for and during revision

There are some basic principles here:

- ideally, notes should be made as soon as possible after a lecture when the information is still fresh in the mind, but life's distractions make a mockery of this fine ideal, and so the disadvantage of not having good notes can be turned to advantage by using note preparation as a form of revision
- revision notes should be as brief and concise as possible, and lecture notes are usually not brief and concise
- heavy textbooks, no matter how heavy and gorgeously plumaged, do not automatically transfer their contents to the buyer's brain on purchase, and the student with time at a premium does not have the time for assimilation of such books
- revision notes, especially in an emergency, should be portable and their information instantly accessible for honest use during train rides etc.

With these principles in mind, a method is suggested below which on more than one occasion has saved the author's skin, and which may suit some readers.

A suggested method of compiling notes for revision purposes

Equipment needed (apart from pens, pencils erasers etc): filing cards of dimensions 8 inches by 5 inches (20 × 13 cm approximately). These are available from stationery shops and some supermarkets. All the information needed about a hormone, its mechanisms, uses etc will be contained on one of these cards. The card system can also be used for making tables, diagrams and graphs. The overriding principle is to simplify, summarise and reduce the volume of notes, and it is hoped that some students will find this suggestion helpful.

Some readers may ask why the author didn't save them the trouble by preparing the cards, but that would defeat the purpose, since the process is a powerful form of learning. A vital part of this learning method is actively to find the information relevant to a given heading, and in any event this book does contain emergency rations. Furthermore, for some reason publishers don't publish revision cards. An example of a revision card is shown in Figure 1.1.

At the end of each chapter is a quiz. This follows the course of each chapter closely and is intended as a supplement to each chapter and a reminder of the contents. The questions are for the most part True/False choices, and there are some gentle traps. It is hoped that the tests will, in the main, reinforce the information in the chapter.

Hormone: Insulin:
Source: Pancreatic islet β-cells
Release is stimulated by:
- Glucose mainly
- Carbohydrates
- Most amino acids
- Fatty acids, ketones
  Main actions: Anabolic, by:

- Removal of glucose from the circulation by uptake into cells
- Promotion of glucose ➔ glycogen+lipids
- Promotion of fatty acids ➔ lipids
- Promotion of amino acid uptake ➔ liver and muscle for new protein synthesis

Other actions of insulin:

- Growth factor in mammary gland
- Stimulation of membrane ATPase in lymphocytes

Insulin deficiency (diabetes) results in:
  Hyperglycaemia (raised blood glucose) which results in a catabolic state since cells are deprived of an energy source, and cells start breaking down their constituents for fuel by:

- Glycogenolysis (glycogen breakdown)
- Gluconeogenensis from protein and fat, which results in:
- Ketone production ➔ bloodstream and associated acidosis
which all result in:
- Acidosis, + vasodilation & hypothermia
- Body wasting
- Excess glucose ➔ urine, with associated dehydration
- Coma and death if left untreated

 Other side of card

Types of diabetes mellitus
- **Type 1 diabetes** (juvenile onset diabetes)
- **Type 2 diabetes** (adult onset diabetes (*now a misnomer with modern obesity in children*)

Type 1 diabetes:
  Cause: Destruction of pancreatic β islet cells, possibly by autoimmune disease

Treatment
- Parenteral (S.C.) human insulin
- Carefully regulated diet

Types of insulin
- **Short-acting (Soluble)**
  e.g. Humulin; Human actrapid; Insulin lispro
- **Intermediate-acting**
  e.g. Insulin Zn suspension; biphasic isophane.
- **Long-acting**
  e.g. Protamine Zn insulin (PZI); Human ultratard

Overdosage with insulin causes:
- Decrease in blood sugar dizziness, tremor, sweating + symptoms of drunkenness ➔ coma and death if untreated with insulin or glucagon

Type 2 diabetes [Non-insulin-dependent (NIDDM);adult onset]
  Caused by obesity, high sugar intake ➔ islet exhaustion ➔ reduced responsiveness to glucose

Possible clinical consequences if untreated (similar to those of juvenile onset)
- Myocardial infarction   • Vascular disease
- Renal failure   • Retinopathy

Treatment
  Reduce patient's weight with diet; cut down sugar, carbohydrate, saturated animal fat intake

Oral hypoglycaemic agents
- **Sulphonylureas**
  glipizide   gliquadone
  gliclazide,   tolbutamide
- **Metformin**
  Thiazolidinediones
  pioglitazone rosiglitazone
- **Prandial glucose regulators**
  nateglinide repaglinide
- **Acarbose**

Figure 1.1 Example of a revision card.

Case history

This is an account of an experience of a failure to prepare adequately for a university examination. The student is painfully well known to the writer but for obvious reasons must remain anonymous. During his first year at university this student was so consumed by the novelty of personal freedom and the social possibilities that he did no work whatsoever, and two weeks before the finals realised he had taken most of his notes in lectures while asleep. He therefore embarked on a strict course of study consisting of no sleep, very strong black coffee and the attempted assimilation of several weighty tomes borrowed from the university library.

On the morning of the examination the student awoke, caught a bus to the examination and on alighting at his bus stop discovered that the bus was under attack from the rear by an alien space ship. The student immediately attacked the space ship and tore it to pieces with his bare hands, after which he was carried in triumph to a palace and given a bed in a room thronged with cheering crowds.

After his recovery the student was told that he went to his examination wearing his pyjamas and after alighting at the bus terminus he ran to the bus immediately behind and started kicking it. He was taken to hospital by ambulance where he required rehydration, nutritional therapy and bed rest. He also learned that he had gone to the examination two days after it was actually scheduled.

Further reading

- Greenstein B and Wood D. *Endocrine Systems at a Glance* (2e). Oxford: Blackwell Science, 2005.

2 Endocrine systems overview

Learning objectives
Basic definitions
Major endocrine organs
Major endocrine-sensitive metabolic systems
Major endocrine glands and hormones
Endocrinology of lipoprotein metabolism
Major endocrine disorders

Learning objectives

- Know the basic definitions
- Know the approximate anatomical location of the major endocrine glands and major functions of their endocrine hormones
- Have some knowledge of major diseases associated with hormonal excess or deficiency

Basic definitions

- *Endocrinology*: the science of ductless glands and their hormones
- *Hormone*: a chemical messenger released from the cell that produces it
- *Endocrine hormones*: hormones produced by ductless glands
- *Autocrine hormone*: a hormone that acts on the cell that secretes it
- *Paracrine hormone*: a hormone that acts on cells neighbouring the cells that secrete it
- *Endocrine hormone*: a hormone that acts on distant sites, which is carried to them usually in the bloodstream
- *Pheromonal hormone*: a hormone released into the atmosphere

Major endocrine organs (*see* Figure 2.1)

- Hypothalamus
- Pituitary gland
- Thyroid gland
- Parathyroid gland
- Parafollicular cells
- Adrenal gland
- Endocrine pancreas
- Gastrointestinal tract (GIT)
- Kidney

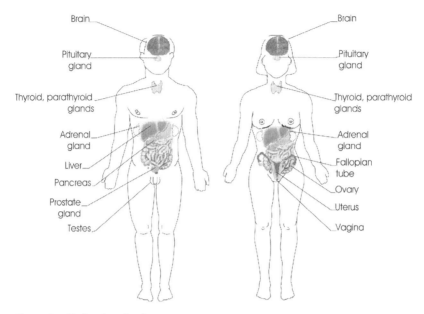

Figure 2.1 Endocrine glands.

- Ovary
- Testes
- Liver
- Blood elements
- Adipocytes
- Skin

Major endocrine-sensitive metabolic systems

- Lipoprotein
- Mineral

Major endocrine glands and hormones

Brain

Hypothalamus

- *Corticotrophin-releasing hormone* (CRH)
- *Gonadotrophin-releasing hormone* (GnRH)
- *Growth-hormone-releasing hormone* (GHRH)
- *Growth hormone-inhibitory hormone* (somatostatin)
- *Dopamine* (prolactin-inhibitory factor)

- *Oxytocin* ⎫ Stored in and released from
- *Vasopressin*[1] ⎬ the posterior pituitary gland
- *Thyrotrophin-releasing hormone* (TRH)

Pineal gland
- *Melatonin*: may control some body rhythms

Pituitary gland
Anatomical situation – at the base of the brain in the sella turcica (*see* Figure 2.2(a)).

Anterior pituitary
- *Corticotrophin* (ACTH, adrenocorticotrophic hormone): releases adrenal cortex hormones
- *Growth hormone* (GH): promotes skeletal, muscle growth
- *Luteinising hormone* (LH): ruptures the ripe Graafian follicle; releases ovarian estrogens and testicular testosterone
- *Follicle-stimulating hormone* (FSH): promotes follicular growth, spermatogenesis
- *Prolactin*: promotes milk production
- *Thyrotrophin* (TSH, thyroid-stimulating hormone): promotes thyroid hormone production and release

All these hormones are carried to the anterior pituitary gland in the blood portal system (see Figure 2.2(b)).

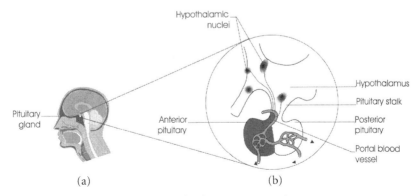

Figure 2.2 (a) The pituitary gland; (b) the pituitary portal system.

[1] Vasopressin and oxytocin are somewhat unusual since they are produced in the brain but secreted into the circulation from the pituitary gland.

Posterior pituitary
- *Oxytocin*: stimulates milk release, uterine contractions
- *Vasopressin*: promotes water reabsorption in the kidney tubule

Intermediate pituitary lobe
- *Melanocyte-stimulating hormone*: stimulates pigment production, possibly regulates some bodily rhythms

Thyroid gland

- Anatomical situation in humans is in front of the trachea; produces thyroxine (T_4) and tri-iodothyronine (T_3) in follicle cells, which powerfully concentrate iodine (*see* p. 160).
- *Parathyroid glands* are embedded in the thyroid gland and produce parathyroid hormone (parathormone; PTH) which is involved in calcium and phosphate regulation (*see* p. 182).
- *Parafollicular cells* are embedded in the thyroid between follicles and produce calcitonin, which inhibits calcium resorption from bone (*see* p. 191).

Adrenal glands

The adrenal glands are situated above the kidneys and consist of an outer cortex, which synthesises *glucocorticoid* and *mineralocorticoid steroids* and an inner medulla which produces epinephrine (adrenaline) and norepinephrine (noradrenaline) (*see* p. 135).

The endocrine pancreas

This consists of islet cells in the exocrine pancreas, which lies across the upper posterior abdominal wall (*see* Figure 2.1).

Nomenclature note

Exocrine means glands with ducts e.g. salivary glands

Pancreatic hormones
- *Insulin*: promotes glucose removal from the bloodstream (*see* p. 149)
- *Glucagon*: increases glucose concentrations in the bloodstream (*see* p. 156)
- *Pancreatic polypeptide*: function unknown
- *Somatostatin*: paracrine regulator of insulin and glucagon release?

The gastrointestinal tract

This is the largest endocrine gland; its hormones are mainly peptides.

- *Cholecystokinin* (CCK): releases glucagon, stimulates pancreatic enzymes, contracts the gall bladder
- *Gastric inhibitory peptide*: enhances insulin release from the pancreas during hyperglycaemia
- *Gastrin*: promotes HCl release, gastric mucosa growth
- *Gastrin-releasing peptide*: releases gastrin
- *Ghrelin*: promotes feeding behaviour, stimulates GH release from the anterior pituitary
- *Motilin*: contracts upper gut muscles
- *Neurotensin*: function unknown
- *Secretin*: stimulates HCO_3^- release from the pancreas, potentiates CCK action
- *Substance P: function unknown*
- *Vasoactive intestinal peptide* (VIP): promotes descending gut relaxation?

> *Note*: the GIT produces many peptide hormones; possibly not all have been identified and the functional significance of many already identified is still unclear or unknown.

Kidney

- *Erythropoietin*: stimulates red blood cell production in the bone marrow (*see* p. 39)
- *Renin*: enzyme splitting angiotensinogen into angiotensin I (*see* p. 124)

Ovary

- *Estrogens*
- *Progesterone*
- *Relaxin*: a polypeptide that softens the cervix during labour in some animals; promotes water uptake and glycogen synthesis in the uterine myometrium (*see* p. 82)
- *Inhibin*: a glycoprotein produced also by the testis and the fetoplacental unit, which inhibits FSH production in the anterior pituitary gland

Placenta

Interface between mother and developing fetus; secretes several hormones, notably:

- *Chorionic gonadotrophin* (CG; HCG, H = human): action similar to that of LH
- *Placental lactogen* (PL) – role unknown (*see* p. 82)

- *Estriol*: role unknown, but blood levels in the mother are a marker of fetal development
- *Progesterone*: essential for pregnancy (*see* p. 82)

Testis

- *Testosterone*: anabolic hormone of male sexual and aggressive behaviour, and fertility (*see* p. 112)
- *Inhibin*: inhibits FSH production in the anterior pituitary gland (*see* p. 71)
- *Fetal Müllerian regression (inhibiting) factor*: dedifferentiates the Müllerian duct (*see* p. 54)

Adipocytes

Adipocytes (fat cells) produce the peptide hormone *leptin,* which is important in the control of feeding and energy expenditure, and is implicated in obesity.

Endocrinology of lipoprotein metabolism

Circulating lipoproteins and the ratio of low-density lipoprotein (LDL): high-density lipoprotein (HDL) together with the negative feedback effects on the LDL receptor determine the concentrations of circulating cholesterol and the risk of atherosclerosis. The system is therefore highly analogous to other hormonal feedback systems and brings this topic into the sphere of cardiovascular endocrinology.

Circulating blood elements

- *White blood cells*: release peptides, e.g. cytokines

Skin

- *Vitamin D*: also released by the liver and kidney; now considered to have hormonal status (*see* p. 183)

Major endocrine disorders

Figure 2.3 summarises the sources of endocrine disorders.

Hypothalamus/pituitary

Lesions present with symptoms including:

- hyper- or hyposecretion of pituitary hormones (early symptoms)
- visual loss (due to pressure on optic nerve; a later symptom)
- enlargement of the sella turcica (depression in the sphenoid bone that houses the pituitary gland; a later symptom).

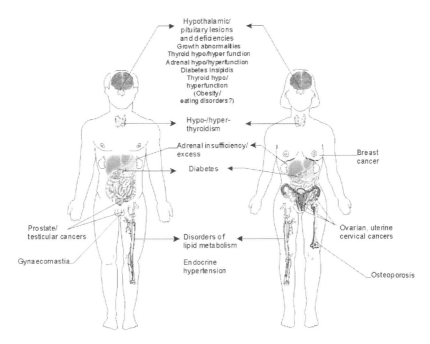

Figure 2.3 Endocrine-related disorders.

Causes of hypothalamic–pituitary dysfunction

- *Hypersecreting pituitary adenoma* (adults): most commonly excess *prolactin* secretion; hypersecretion of growth hormone and ACTH can cause acromegaly and Cushing's syndrome respectively
- *Craniopharyngiomas*: more prevalent in children; brain tumour derived from Rathke's pouch, an embryonic structure contributing to development of the pituitary gland; other hypothalamic tumours; consequences include diabetes insipidus, low circulating GH levels and delayed puberty (*see* p. 9)
- *Infarction*: ischaemic damage to the pituitary gland through failure of perfusion with arterial blood
- *Hypopituitarism*: invasive, space-occupying tumours in the sella turcica
- *Severe head trauma*
- *Iatrogenic*: radiation therapy, chemical therapy or surgery may cause inadvertent hypothalamic or pituitary damage causing e.g. diabetes insipidus, which is caused by failure to produce vasopressin (ADH)
- *Idiopathic*: no discernible cause

> *Clinical note*: circulating prolactin levels are often an indicator of pituitary dysfunction.

Treatment summary

> *Study note*: all treatments mentioned below are dealt with in more detail in relevant chapters.

Pituitary adenomas
- *Prolactinoma*: suppress prolactin secretion with a dopamine agonist; irradiation; surgery
- *GH-secreting adenoma*: suppress GH secretion with octreotide acetate (analogue of somatostatin); irradiation; transphenoidal microsurgery
- *ACTH-secreting adenoma (Cushing's disease)*: transphenoidal resection of adenoma; supplementary drugs e.g. ketoconazole, aminoglutethimide
- *Thyrotrophin-secreting adenoma* (often a large tumour): transphenoidal microsurgery; octreotide; partial thyroidectomy may be necessary to control thyrotoxicosis

Craniopharyngiomas, iatrogenic or head injury
These may cause diabetes insipidus (*see* above).

- *Drug treatment with desmopressin*, an analogue of vasopressin (*see* p. 121)

Thyroid (see p. 23)
Hypothyroidism
- Primary hypothyroidism (thyroid failure; *see* p. 165)
- Hypothyroidism secondary to pituitary TSH deficit (*see* p. 164)

Hyperthyroidism (not a comprehensive list)
- Diffuse toxic goitre (Graves' disease; *see* p. 165)
- Thyrotoxicosis factitia
- Subacute thyroiditis
- Toxic adenoma
- Toxic multinodular goitre

Treatment summary
- *Hypothyroidism*: drug treatment with thyroxine
- *Hyperthyroidism*: drugs include methimazole, propylthiouracil; radioactive iodine therapy; subtotal thyroidectomy; propranolol to control cardiac symptoms

Growth disorders

> *Clinical note*: stature may be short or tall through normal genetic factors, or constitutional through phenotypic variation from accepted norms of pace of growth within a given population. These are generally considered non-endocrine growth determinants.

Endocrine-related short stature
- Deficiency of GHRH secretion through idiopathic growth hormone deficiency or hypothalamic tumour
- Deficiency of GH secretion due to pituitary tumours, dysplasia (abnormal pituitary development), surgery or trauma (*see* p. 43)
- Laron's dwarfism through GH receptor defect
- Dwarfism through low insulin-like growth factor-1 (IGF-1) production or resistance to IGF-1
- Prolonged treatment with glucocorticoids or Cushing's syndrome during growth phase
- Psychosocial dwarfism through child abuse which causes functional hypopituitarism and low circulating GH – reversible if child is removed from the abusive environment

Endocrine-related tall stature in children and adults
- Pituitary giantism is caused by a GH-producing pituitary adenoma before bone epiphyseal closure (*see* p. 37)
- Precocious puberty may bring an increased rate of growth through abnormally high release of androgens or estrogens, resulting in premature epiphyseal closure and a tall child but a short adult (*see* p. 62)
- Thyrotoxicosis in children causes advanced bone age, resulting, as with precocious puberty, in a tall child but a short adult (*see* p. 164)
- Moderately diabetic women may give birth to abnormally large babies

Treatment summary
- *Growth hormone deficiency*: growth hormone replacement therapy until epiphyseal closure

Adrenal disorders
Adrenocortical insufficiency
- *Primary adrenocortical insufficiency* (Addison's disease)
- *Secondary adrenocortical insufficiency*: usually caused by corticosteroid therapy or, less frequently, by hypothalamic or pituitary tumours

Adrenal over-secretion
- *Cushing's syndrome*: consequence of chronic glucocorticoid excess (*see* p. 33)
- *Virilisation and hirsutism* due to excess androgen secretion by the adrenal cortex (*see* p. 51); in children causes precocious puberty
- *Phaeochromocytoma*: abnormal secretion of epinephrine and norepinephrine by an adrenal medulla tumour (*see* p. 172)

Treatment summary
- *Acute Addisonian crisis and maintenance*: drug treatment with glucocorticoids and mineralocorticoids; fluid replacement; maintenance for life on these drugs (*see* p. 142)
- *Cushing's syndrome*: surgery to remove tumour; drug treatment to reduce glucocorticoid/mineralocorticoid levels; aim is to reduce ACTH secretion from the anterior pituitary
- *Virilisation and hirsutism*: if caused by CNS or pituitary tumours, treat with a GnRH analogue, which suppresses the production of gonadotrophins in the hypothalamus–anterior pituitary axis

Endocrine hypertension

Causes
- *Phaeochromocytoma*: catecholamine-secreting adrenal medullary or ectopic tumour; *treatment*: alpha-adrenergic antagonists and surgery
- *Primary aldosteronism*: abnormally high aldosterone secretion by adrenal glomerulosa hyperplasia or tumour or, more rarely, idiopathic, resulting in activation of the renin–aldosterone system; *treatment*: for an adrenal tumour, unilateral adrenalectomy or adenoma removal
- *Excess deoxycorticosterone (DOC) production*: due to enzyme deficiencies results in deficient cortisol production; *treatment*: glucocorticoid replacement therapy
- *Cushing's syndrome*: appears to cause hypertension through glucocorticoid over-stimulation of hepatic angiotensinogen production and inhibition of various vasodilator mechanisms; *treatment*: see p. 145
- *Hypertension mediated by the renin–angiotensin–aldosterone system*; *treatment* is mainly surgical e.g. transluminal angioplasty

Disorders of lipid metabolism

- *Primary hyperlipidaemias*:
  - primary hypercholesterolaemia (without hypertriglyceridaemia)
  - primary hypertriglyceridaemia (without hypercholesterolaemia)
  - primary mixed (or combined) hyperlipidaemia

- *Secondary hyperlipidaemias* are caused by, e.g. alcoholism, cholestasis, chronic renal failure, diabetes mellitus, high doses of estrogens, hypothyroidism, liver disease, obesity or smoking

Treatments
- Statins
- Fibrates
- Anion exchange resins
- Cholesterol absorption inhibitors
- Nicotinic acid
- Omega-3 triglycerides (fish oils)

Obesity

Obesity is associated with potentially life-threatening metabolic and cardiovascular disorders, including diabetes mellitus and thromboembolic disease. A serious sign of the growing problem is the appearance of obesity and type 2 diabetes in young children. It may be an important endocrine condition, since a circulating hormone, leptin, which is released by adipocytes, is involved in the control of feeding behaviour. Other endocrine hormones which, through inappropriate action, might contribute to obesity are growth hormone, glucagon, thyroxine, insulin and the adrenal glucocorticoids, growth hormone, insulin, glucagon, all of which play an important part in the regulation of glucose flows and therefore in the integration of fat, carbohydrate and protein metabolism.

Treatment
There are no accredited drug treatments for obesity yet, and treatment is currently population education and tighter control over the promotion of fattening foods.

Disorders of calcium

- Vitamin D deficiency and compensatory hyperparathyroidism
- Primary hyperparathyroidism
- Malignancy-associated hypercalcaemia
- Iatrogenic hypercalcaemia
- Hypoparathyroidism
- Pseudohypoparathyroidism

Treatments
Treatments depend on the cause of hyper- or hypocalcaemia.

- *Hypercalcaemia*: treatments include rehydration, correction of renal impairment and induction of saline diuresis
- *Acute hypocalcaemia*: calcium chloride IV (intravenous) to treat tetany;

secure airways if stridor (breathing noises indicating airways obstruction) is heard

> *Safety note*: before giving calcium IV, determine if the patient is on digoxin, since digoxin toxicity is enhanced by calcium.

- *Chronic hypocalcaemia*: treatment aims to maintain serum calcium at about 8.5–9.2 mg/dl, and keep patients free of symptoms. Oral calcium plus vitamin D are prescribed

> *Safety note*: monitor serum calcium regularly to avoid suppression of PTH release and subsequent loss of its hypocalcaemic effect, which could result in nephrocalcinosis, nephrolithiasis and chronic renal insufficiency.

Disorders of bone remodelling

- *Osteoporosis*: loss of bone mass
- *Osteomalacia*: defective bone matrix mineralisation
- *Paget's disease of bone*: accelerated rates of bone turnover, causing gross deformity of bone

Reproductive disorders

Female disorders

Disorders and failures of ovarian and menstrual function and treatments

- *Delayed puberty*: amenorrhoea (failure to begin menstruation)
- *Precocious puberty*: abnormally early development of reproductive organs and function; treatment aims to suppress this, e.g. with chronic GnRH administration
- *Menstrual cycle disturbances*: amenorrhoea in adults, which may have one of several causes (*see* p. 71); treatment depends on diagnosis of the underlying cause
- *Anovulatory bleeding*
- *Excess androgen secretion*: treatment is aimed at the amenorrhoea and hirsutism (*see* p. 76)

Interventions in normal female reproductive processes

- *Oral contraception*: routine drug treatment of healthy women to block ovulation (*see* p. 90)

- *Abortion*: termination of pregnancy, either physically or using drugs
- *Menopause*: a normal age-related cessation of ovarian function which is often accompanied by distressing symptoms; it is now regarded in several societies as a disorder and is treated with various combinations of low-dose estrogens, androgens and progesterone (*see* p. 101)

Male disorders
- *Disorders of male sexual function*
- *Klinefelter's syndrome*: extra X chromosome causes Leydig cell dysgenesis
- *Leydig cell aplasia*: failure of Leydig cell development causes male pseudohermaphroditism and ambiguous genitalia
- *Bilateral anorchia*: absence of testes
- *Cryptorchidism*: failure of testes to descend from the genital ridge during development
- *Male infertility*: blanket term encompassing all causes of failure to produce spermatozoa capable of fertilising the ovum
- *Gynaecomastia*: breast development in males

Treatments may involve surgery and hormone replacement regimes.

Endocrine-related cancer
- Breast, cervical, ovarian and uterine cancers and estrogen involvement
- Testicular and prostate cancer and androgen involvement

Disorders of puberty
- *Absent or delayed puberty*: no signs of puberty by age 13 in girls or age 14 in boys
- *Precocious puberty*: appearance of secondary sexual characteristics before the age of 8 in girls and before the age of 9 in boys

Causes of delayed puberty
- Hypogonadotrophic hypogonadism
- Hypergonadotrophic hypogonadism

Treatment of delayed puberty
Treatment of delayed puberty depends on the diagnosis, and includes sex hormone replacement, treatment with growth hormone if appropriate, and psychological support.

Causes of precocious puberty
- Premature activation of the hypothalamus–anterior pituitary axis
- Ectopic secretion of gonadotrophins or sex hormones

Treatment of precocious puberty

Treatment of precocious puberty depends on the diagnosed cause, and may include surgery to remove tumours and drug therapy including:

- *chronic GnRH treatment*, which desensitises anterior pituitary gonadotrophes to GnRH (*see* p. 63)
- *progestational steroids*, which block anterior pituitary gonadotrophin treatment by negative feedback
- *sex steroid antagonists*, e.g. the androgen receptor antagonist cyproterone acetate.

Diabetes

- *Insulin-dependent diabetes mellitus* (IDDM): caused by loss of insulin-producing islet cells; treated with insulin
- *Non-insulin-dependent diabetes mellitus* (NIDDM): characterised by tissue resistance to insulin, defective insulin release or defective insulin or pro-insulin; causes are unknown but may include obesity; *treatment* aims to supplement with insulin and lower blood glucose with oral hypoglycaemic drugs.

Clinical note: hypoglycaemia is clinically low blood glucose and may result from

- inappropriate use of or inadvertent overdose with insulin
- drugs such as alcohol
- inborn errors of carbohydrate metabolism
- obsessive fasting or be of unknown cause.

Chapter 2 quiz

Answer T (true) or F (false)

1 Endocrine hormones are produced by ductless glands ☐
2 Paracrine hormones act on cells that produce them ☐
3 The pituitary gland is situated below the sella turcica ☐
4 ACTH releases adrenal medullary hormones ☐
5 Corticotrophin releases ACTH ☐
6 FSH promotes LH secretion ☐
7 The thyroid gland is located in front of the trachea ☐
8 Calcitonin promotes calcium resorption from bone ☐
9 Insulin promotes glucose removal from the blood ☐
10 CCK releases insulin from the pancreas ☐
11 Ghrelin promotes feeding behaviour ☐
12 Motilin contracts upper gut muscles ☐
13 Erythropoietin promotes red blood cell production ☐
14 Relaxin is produced by the ovary ☐
15 High HDL is a risk factor for atherosclerosis ☐
16 The term iatrogenic describes treatment-induced disease ☐
17 Vitamin D is not produced by the kidney ☐
18 Craniopharyngiomas are brain tumours ☐
19 Prolactinomas can be treated with a dopamine antagonist ☐
20 Thyrotoxicosis is caused by excessive thyroid secretion ☐
21 Laron's dwarfism is the result of a GH receptor defect ☐
22 Cushing's syndrome is due to excessive androgen production ☐
23 Phaeochromocytoma is a catecholamine-secreting tumour ☐
24 Endocrine hypertension may result from low DOC production ☐
25 Obesity is associated with type 2 diabetes ☐
26 Digoxin toxicity is enhanced by calcium ☐
27 Osteomalacia is excessive bone mineralisation ☐
28 Chronic GnRH treatment promotes gonadotrophin secretion ☐
29 Precocious puberty may be treated with progestational steroids ☐
30 Insulin-dependent diabetes is treated with oral hypoglycaemic drugs ☐

A Insulin:
- Is released from islet cells in the pancreas ☐
- Inhibits glucose uptake into cells ☐
- Release is enhanced by gastric inhibitory peptide ☐
- Release is impaired in obesity ☐
- Is used in insulin-independent diabetes mellitus ☐
- Is taken orally in tablet form ☐

B The anterior pituitary gland:
- Secretes oxytocin and vasopressin ☐
- Secretes ACTH under the control of CRH ☐
- Controls thyroid function by secreting TRH ☐
- Secretion of LH is inhibited by progesterone ☐

C The hypothalamus:
- Secretes somatostatin ☐
- Synthesises oxytocin and vasopressin ☐
- Can develop tumours affecting growth ☐
- Controls anterior pituitary endocrine function through nervous connections ☐

D The anterior pituitary gland secretes:
- ACTH ☐
- Somatostatin ☐
- Ghrelin ☐
- Dopamine ☐

E Hypothalamic–pituitary dysfunction in adults is usually due to:
- Craniopharyngiomas ☐
- Infarction of pituitary blood vessels ☐
- Hypersecreting pituitary adenomas ☐

F Hyperprolactinaemia:
- Can be treated with a dopamine agonist ☐
- Is under-secretion of prolactin ☐
- Is a possible indicator of a pituitary problem ☐

G Endocrine-related short stature:
- May be due to prolonged treatment with glucocorticoids ☐
- Is a result of precocious puberty ☐
- May be caused by a GH mutation ☐
- Is treated with GH until epiphyseal closure ☐

H Endocrine hypertension may result from:
- Phaeochromocytoma ☐
- Deficient DOC production ☐
- Abnormally high aldosterone secretion ☐
- Cushing's syndrome ☐
- Primary aldosteronism ☐

3 Summary of basic cellular mechanisms

Learning objectives
Relevance of mechanisms to basic and clinical
   endocrinology
Mechanism summary
Basic sites of hormone action
Receptors

Learning objectives

- Appreciate the relevance of basic cellular mechanisms to the patient and the scientist
- Be acquainted with the meaning of the mechanisms listed below
- Know the meanings of the terms describing the sites of hormone action
- Be able to distinguish the difference between extra- and intracellular receptors with examples

Relevance of mechanisms to basic and clinical endocrinology

- Receptor studies contribute to new drug development e.g. receptor antagonists such as tamoxifen, which blocks the action of estrogens and is used to treat estrogen-responsive breast cancer.
- Knowledge of cellular mechanisms contributes to an understanding of the cellular events underlying hormone action, e.g. the study of iodide uptake into the thyroid cell and the mechanisms resulting in thyroglobulin production and release. This leads to an understanding of the actions of thyroid-stimulating hormone (TSH) and to the development of drugs that interfere with these processes and that are used to treat hyperthyroidism.
- The discovery of intracellular second messengers which mediate the actions of hormones increases our understanding of how these hormones exert their effects on the cell and therefore the whole body's response to the hormone. For example, the discovery of *cyclic AMP*, which is a second messenger for the hormone epinephrine, explains how the actions of one molecule of epinephrine on a cell are amplified through the stimulation of several molecules of cyclic AMP in the cell. The discovery also explains how stimulant drugs such as aminophylline cause dilation of bronchioles

in asthma by blocking the phosphodiesterase enzyme that normally breaks down cyclic AMP.
- Studies of hormone biosynthesis may lead to an understanding of the aetiology of certain endocrine disorders such as hirsutism, amenorrhoea, acne and virilism of the external genitalia, which is caused by deficiency of the enzyme 11-β-hydroxylase in the steroid biosynthetic pathway.

Mechanism summary

Enzyme-mediated chemical reactions

- *Biosynthesis*: e.g. proteins from amino acids (anabolic)
- *Biodegradation*: e.g. protein breakdown to amino acids (catabolic)
- *Biotransformation*: e.g. carbohydrate conversion to fat; neurotransmitter biosynthesis from precursors

Physical mechanisms

- *Non-covalent protein binding*: e.g. ligand–receptor binding or substrate–enzyme binding
- *Solute and solvent movement* within and between compartments:
  - *diffusion* (e.g. steroids across all biological membranes)
  - *osmosis* (e.g. process of cell shrinkage and swelling)
  - *phagocytosis* (cell 'swallows' another particle) and *pinocytosis* (ingestion of fluid); both are examples of *endocytosis*, when substances are taken into cells without having to cross membranes
  - *hormone transport in the circulation*: free and protein-bound (e.g. cortisol bound to corticosteroid-binding globulin (CBG); sex hormones bound to sex hormone-binding globulin (SHBG))
  - *facilitated transport*: e.g. glucose transport into the cell
  - *active transport*: active transport across membranes, uses ATP for energy and therefore can pump against a concentration gradient, e.g. ion channels such as the Na^+/K^+ ATPase pump

Energy transduction

- *Electrical impulse $\rightarrow$ neurotransmitter release. Mechanisms of transduction are unknown but probably a combination of chemical, physical and electrical energy*
- *Ligand–receptor binding $\rightarrow$ membrane enzyme activation or inhibition $\rightarrow$ cellular response, e.g. epinephrine–receptor binding $\rightarrow$ membrane adenylate cyclase activation $\rightarrow$ intracellular cyclic AMP synthesis $\rightarrow$ cellular response*
- *Chemical reactions $\rightarrow$ chemical products + heat $\rightarrow$ temperature maintenance*
- *Enzyme catalysis*: conformational changes in enzyme proteins induced by substrate binding $\rightarrow$ chemical reactions and product synthesis

- *Neurosecretion*: a hormone-secreting neurone, e.g. a GnRH neurone in the hypothalamus, is activated and transports GnRH to its terminal on blood vessels of the portal system. GnRH is carried to the anterior pituitary where it binds to its GnRH receptor on gonadotrophs, which in turn release LH and FSH into the general circulation

Basic sites of hormone action

- *Autocrine*: the hormone acts on the cell that released it e.g. IGF-1 on tumour cells
- *Paracrine*: the hormone acts on neighbouring cells e.g. beta-cells of the pancreas release insulin, which inhibits glucagon release from neighbouring pancreatic A cells
- *Endocrine*: the hormone travels in the circulation to distal organs, e.g. adipose cells release leptin, which travels to the hypothalamus in the brain to suppress appetite
- *Neuroendocrine*: the hormone is released from a neurone and acts on neighbouring cells or is released into blood vessels, e.g. GnRH
- *Pheromonal*: the hormone is released into the atmosphere e.g. bombykol from the female silk moth *Bombyx mori*

Receptors

> **Definition**
>
> Receptors are macromolecular components of the cell that selectively recognise and non-covalently bind substances, usually termed *ligands*.

The binding reaction initiates a cascade of reactions, usually starting with a conformational change in the receptor, resulting in intermediate physical and chemical cellular changes ending in the cellular response to the binding reaction. Receptors may be:

- extracellular
- intracellular

Extracellular receptors

Extracellular receptors are situated on the cell membrane (*see* Figure 3.1). Generally, they have three principal domains:

- *extracellular domain*: selectively recognises and binds chemicals, e.g. epinephrine, insulin, glucagon and the gonadotrophins LH, FSH and prolactin, in the extracellular space
- *intramembrane domain*: e.g. the cyclic adenylate system, the inositol

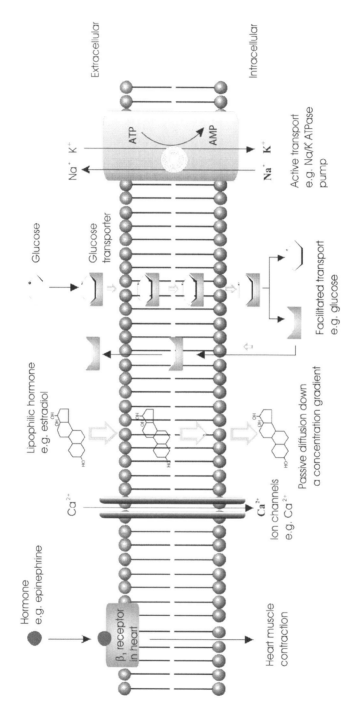

Figure 3.1 Membrane-mediated events.

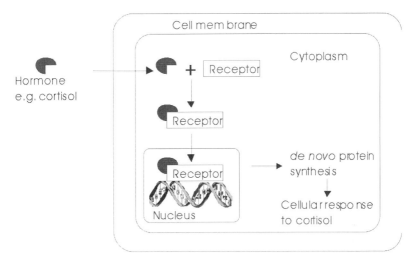

Figure 3.2 Intracellular receptors.

phosphate system or ion channels, which transduce the binding reaction into a physical or chemical response

- *intracellular domain*: transduces the intramembrane response into a physical or chemical response.

Intracellular receptors

Intracellular receptors bind to hormones after they have penetrated the cell membrane, e.g. the lipophilic (fat-soluble) steroid hormones such as estradiol, progesterone, testosterone, thyroid hormone and vitamin D. After the hormone binds to the receptor, the complex attaches itself to the nuclear DNA and, generally, switches on selective mRNA synthesis (*see* Figure 3.2).

Neurotransmitter actions

When the nerve impulse arrives at the presynaptic nerve terminal, it usually stimulates migration of vesicles (packets) of neurotransmitter to the cell membrane, where they release neurotransmitter molecules into the synaptic cleft (*see* Figure 3.3). The neurotransmitter targets are:

- *specific receptors on the postsynaptic cell membrane* (usually nerve, muscle or secretory cell), where the response may be excitation or inhibition of the postsynaptic cell; examples include dopamine, which inhibits prolactin release from anterior pituitary cells and 5-HT, which stimulates CRH release from hypothalamic secretory neurones

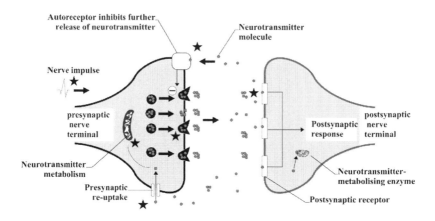

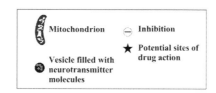

Figure 3.3 The nerve terminal.

- *autoreceptors* on the presynaptic cell, which usually inhibit further release of the neurotransmitter; examples include catecholaminergic α_2-receptors
- *presynaptic neurotransmitter re-uptake* mechanisms on the presynaptic cell membrane, thereby terminating their action; examples include norepinephrine and 5-HT re-uptake mechanisms
- *metabolising enzymes* in the postsynaptic cell, e.g. acetylcholinesterase, which breaks down acetylcholine to choline and acetate.

Other drugs affecting neurotransmission
Local anaesthetics
- Lidocaine
- Procaine

Calcium channel blockers
- Nifedipine
- Verapamil
- Felodipine
- Isradipine

- Diltiazem
- Amlodipine

Potassium channel activators
- Nicorandil

Chapter 3 quiz

Answer T (true) or F (false)

1 Cyclic AMP is a second messenger for epinephrine

2 Aminophylline causes bronchiolar constriction

3 Amenorrhoea can be caused by 11β-hydroxylase deficiency

4 Diffusion requires energy

5 Active transport utilises ATP for energy

6 Glucose is transported into the cell by facilitated transport

7 Neurosecretion is a property of pituitary cells

8 Paracrine cells secrete hormones acting on neighbouring cells

9 GnRH is a neuroendocrine hormone

10 Estradiol works mainly through intracellular receptors

11 Dopamine stimulates prolactin release from the anterior pituitary

12 Acetylcholinesterase inactivates ACh in the presynaptic nerve terminal

13 Presynaptic autoreceptors usually inhibit further release of a neurotransmitter

14 Diltiazem is a potassium channel blocker

4 Control of endocrine hormone release

Learning objectives
Principles of feedback
Endocrine feedback systems
Clinical relevance of biological feedback systems in
 endocrinology
Major sites and causes of endocrine diseases
General principles of diagnostic tests
General principles of treatment
Clinical scenario

Learning objectives

- Understand the basic principles of feedback mechanisms
- Be able to give examples of biological feedback systems in endocrinology
- Know important examples of the relevance of feedback mechanisms in basic and clinical endocrinology and how these may be used as diagnostic tests
- Be able to list general principles of treatment using knowledge of endocrine feedback systems

Principles of feedback

Feedback systems maintain a set point e.g. central heating temperature regulation. Feedback systems may be *positive*, when the parameter controlled e.g. the ovulatory surge of LH from the anterior pituitary (*see* p. 70), is *increased* by the system, or *negative*, when the parameter e.g. ACTH from the anterior pituitary (*see* p. 133), is *decreased* by an increase in circulating cortisol. Biological feedback systems protect the organism from dangerous fluctuations in (e.g.):

- temperature
- blood pressure
- pH
- osmolarity
- hormone levels.

Biological feedback mechanisms also control:

- fertility
- metabolism
- poorly understood cycles of sleep and wakefulness
- circadian and other rhythms.

Essential components of a feedback system (see Figure 4.1)

- A signal
- A transducer
- A sensor
- A responder
- *The signal* may be electrical e.g. an activated circuit, or chemical e.g. a change in pH or an endocrine hormone. The value of the signal, e.g.

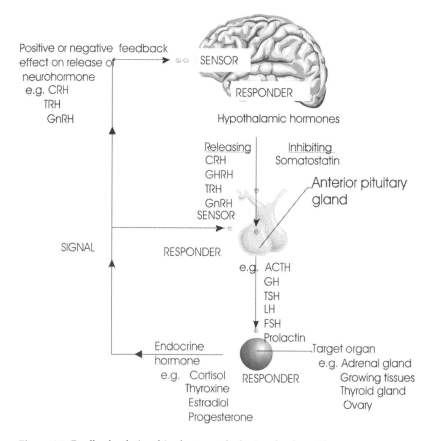

Figure 4.1 Feedback relationships between the brain, glands and hormones.

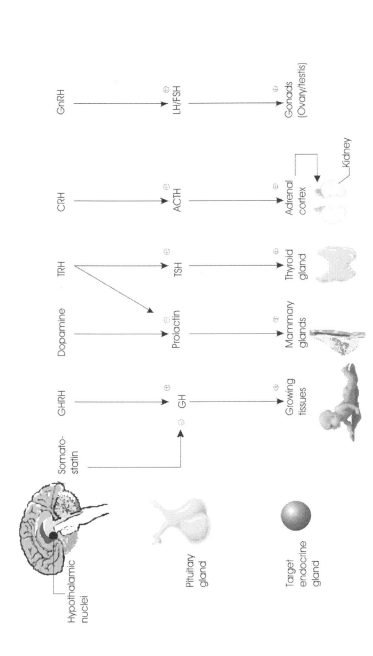

Figure 4.2 Neuroendocrine feedback systems. ACTH, adrenocorticotrophic hormone; CRH, corticotrophin-releasing hormone; FSH, follicle-stimulating hormone; GH, growth hormone; GHRH, growth hormone-releasing hormone; GnRH, gonadotrophin-releasing hormone; TRH, thyrotrophin-releasing hormone; TSH, thyroid-stimulating hormone; LH, luteinising hormone.

temperature, pH or circulating levels of endocrine hormones, may oscillate relatively widely about a set point, or be very tightly controlled e.g. core body temperature

- *The transducer* may be a mechanism that converts physical changes, e.g. magnetic, into another energy form e.g. electricity, or the poorly understood conversion of receptor binding into e.g. neurotransmitter release, enzyme reactions or ion channel opening and closing
- *The sensor* detects a signal, e.g. temperature, pH. In biological systems, the sensor is most commonly a protein receptor, e.g. the cortisol receptor, which binds to a chemical e.g. the endocrine hormone cortisol.

Endocrine feedback systems

Endocrine feedback systems (*see* Figure 4.2) include control of:

- brain and pituitary hormones
- adrenal hormones
- gastrointestinal tract (GIT) hormones
- growth hormones
- sex hormones
- thyroid hormones
- feeding and satiety hormones
- salt and water balance.

Clinical relevance of biological feedback systems in endocrinology

Many endocrine diseases result from disturbances of feedback control systems, and tests of feedback systems are of diagnostic value in, for example:

- acromegaly (*see* p. 37)
- Addison's disease (*see* p. 141)
- Cushing's disease (*see* p. 143)
- diabetes mellitus (*see* p. 151)
- growth disorders (*see* p. 42)
- hypo- or hyperthyroidism (*see* p. 164)
- infertility (*see* p. 112)
- obesity (*see* p. 177).

Major sites and causes of endocrine diseases

- Accidental trauma
- Iatrogenic, e.g. radiotherapy, surgery
- Hypothalamic and pituitary tumours[1]

---

[1] Visual disturbances may occur with hypothalamic or pituitary tumours.

- Absence of hypothalamic growth factors
- Empty sella syndrome
- Ectopic hormone-secreting tumours
- Dietary deficiencies, e.g. iodine
- Peripheral glandular tumours, e.g. adrenal tumours
- Genetic hormone receptor defects, e.g. male testosterone insensitivity, cortisol insensitivity
- Autoimmune disease, e.g. Hashimoto's disease (*see* p. 164)
- Enzyme deficiencies, e.g. 21-hydroxylase deficiency in cortisol biosynthesis
- Extra-glandular causes, e.g. kidney damage leading to defects in vitamin D biosynthesis, resulting in calcium and phosphate imbalances

General principles of diagnostic tests

- Endocrine screening as part of normal check-ups
- Patient history and physical examination, e.g. tissue and bodily changes in acromegaly and Cushing's syndrome
- Use of DNA analysis to diagnose genetically transmitted disease
- Measurement of circulating hormones and other blood tests
- Tests of feedback integrity, e.g. dexamethasone administration to test ACTH response (*see* p. 34)
- Localisation of tumours, using X-ray, magnetic resonance imaging (MRI) and computed tomography (CT) scans

General principles of treatment

- Hormone replacement, e.g. growth hormone in some growth disorders
- Pharmacological blockade of excess hormone production (*see* case history below) or of hormone-receptor interaction, e.g. use of tamoxifen to block estrogen action in estrogen-receptor-positive breast cancer
- Destruction of endocrine tissue using radioactivity, e.g. ^{131}I treatment of some cases of hyperthyroidism
- Surgery to remove hormone-producing tumours (*see* case history below)
- Diet, e.g. in the treatment of type 2 diabetes mellitus (*see* p. 153)

Clinical scenario

Cushing's syndrome results from elevated circulating concentrations of corticosteroids, either endogenous cortisol or administered corticosteroids. In disease, the syndrome is due to either ACTH-dependent or non-ACTH-dependent causes. ACTH-dependent causes can be pituitary or ectopic adenomas which produce ACTH. Non-ACTH-dependent Cushing's syndrome may result from adrenal carcinomas or adenomas which produce large amounts of adrenal steroids.

Case history

Mrs JK, a 38-year-old librarian, was referred to the endocrine clinic at her local hospital by her general practitioner (GP). He queried Cushing's disease when tests revealed a 24-h urinary cortisol of 2355 nmol/24 h and elevated fasting blood glucose of 12 mmol/l. On examination, she presented with hirsutism, scalp hair thinning, abdominal striae (thin streaks on skin) and the characteristic 'buffalo hump' consistent with a redistribution of body fat. She complained of spontaneous bruising, muscle weakness and weight gain despite dieting. Her blood pressure was elevated. Gliclazide 40 mg twice a day was prescribed to treat the high blood glucose. Several endocrine tests were done, including CRH and low and high dexamethasone tests of her adrenal feedback system. An MRI revealed a pituitary adenoma which subsequently was found to be the source of excess ACTH, and the patient was referred for transphenoidal surgery after stabilisation of her various symptoms. Metapyrone was prescribed to reduce circulating cortisol and the gliclazide was stopped when blood glucose levels were normalised.

Note: metapyrone (USA: metyrapone) inhibits the adrenal cortex enzyme β-hyroxylase, which catalyses the final step in the biosynthesis of cortisol. It was used here to prepare the patient for surgery.

Chapter 4 quiz

Answer T (true) or F (false)

A Biofeedback:
- Is a form of nourishment ☐
- Is a biosysytem controlling a set point e.g. hormone levels ☐

B A negative feedback system:
- Increases the value of the set point ☐
- Decreases the value of the set point ☐

C Biofeedback mechanisms control:
- Fertility ☐
- Metabolism ☐
- Human sexual behaviour ☐
- Adrenal hormones ☐
- Salt and water balance ☐

D The components of a biofeedback system include:
- A signal ☐
- A transducer ☐
- A sensor ☐
- A responder ☐

E Can you list at least 8 systems controlled by feedback?

F Name at least 6 diseases caused by disturbances to biofeedback systems

G What are some important general principles of treatment of endocrine diseases?

5 Growth hormone and growth factors

Learning objectives
Growth hormone
Other growth factors

Learning objectives

- Know the main functions of growth hormone (GH)
- Be able to describe briefly where GH is synthesised and how GH release is controlled
- Be able to list the given direct and indirect effects of GH
- Be aware of the main consequences of GH deficiency in adults and children, excess GH, and the treatments
- Read the table of other growth factors

Definition

Growth factors are proteins that activate cellular proliferation and/or cellular differentiation.

Growth hormone

See Figure 5.1.

Functions

- Promotion of growth in children
- Important for maintenance of good physical and mental health in adults

Actions

- *Direct*: by stimulating gluconeogenesis in muscle and lipolysis in fat – therefore GH is diabetogenic since it opposes the actions of insulin (*see* p. 150)
- *Indirect*: by stimulating synthesis of IGF-1 in liver and in bone chondrocytes; IGF-1 in turn stimulates bone growth. GH actions are mediated by a specific membrane GH receptor which activates intracellular kinases

Synthesis and chemistry

GH is synthesised in anterior pituitary somatotroph cells, and is a single-chain 191-amino acid polypeptide.

Control of GH release

GH is released in response to hypothalamic growth hormone-releasing hormone and GH release is inhibited by hypothalamic somatostatin (*see* Figure 5.1(a)).

GH deficiency

GH deficiency is generally caused by hypothalamic–pituitary disorders. In children this causes failure to grow; in adults it causes abnormal metabolism with subsequent imbalances of fat, muscle and bone metabolism. Psychological disturbances include anxiety, mood depression and withdrawal from society.

Treatment of GH deficiency

Treatment of GH deficiency in children is regular treatment with GH until growth is complete.

GH excess

GH excess is usually the result of a pituitary adenoma and results in *gigantism* in children and *acromegaly* in adults. Acromegaly is characterised by:

- enlargement of the lower mandible of the jaw
- coarsening of facial skin (*see* Figure 5.1(b))
- hypertrophy of the heart, kidney and liver connective tissue
- diabetes in some patients through lowered glucose tolerance
- exacerbation of pre-existing heart disease and rheumatism.

Treatment of excess GH

- Surgery or irradiation to remove tumours
- Drugs, e.g. bromocriptine, a dopamine agonist which blocks both GH and prolactin release
- Treatment of any diabetes, rheumatic or cardiovascular symptoms

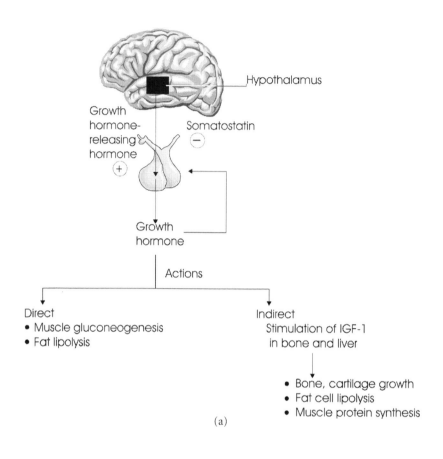

(a)

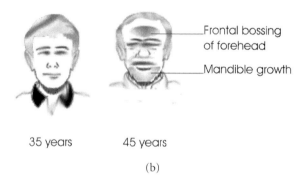

35 years   45 years

(b)

Figure 5.1 (a) Release of growth hormone and actions on tissues; (b) effects of acromegaly on facial configuration. IGF-1, insulin-like growth factor-1.

Other growth factors

Table 5.1 Some other individual growth factors[a]

Growth factor	Source	Activities
Colony-stimulating factors (CSF)	Many types and sources	Proliferation of e.g. pluripotent bone marrow stem cells, macrophages, lymphoid cells, granulocytes
Epidermal growth factor (EGF)	Submaxillary gland	Stimulates proliferation of epithelial, glial and mesenchymal cells; involved in carcinogenesis
Erythropoietin	Kidney	Stimulates differentiation and proliferation of erythrocytes
Fibroblast growth factors (at least 19 subtypes identified)	Many cell types	Stimulates proliferation of e.g. early embryonic mesoderm
Insulin-like growth factor-1 (IGF-1; sometimes called somatomedin C)	Mainly liver	Mediates actions of growth hormone; structurally related to insulin
IGF-2	Mainly in embryonic and neonatal cells	May be a fetal growth factor/hormone
Interleukins 1α and β (IL-1)	Mainly macrophages and various other antigen-presenting cells	Co-stimulation of T and antigen-presenting cells; very important modulator of immune responses
IL-2	Natural killer (NK) and activated thymocyte helper (TH_1) cells	Mediates NK function and proliferation of activated T cells and B cells
IL-3	Activated T cells	Mediates growth of haematopoietic progenitor cells
IL-4	Mast cells and TH_2 cells	Inhibits cytokine production in monocytes and macrophages; mediates eosinophil and mast cell growth and B cell proliferation
IL-5	Mast cells and TH_2 cells	Mediates eosinophil growth and function
IL-6	Several cell types, including antigen-presenting cells, activated TH_2 cells	Acute phase responses; B cell proliferation; synergises with IL-1 and TNF in T cell function; thrombopoiesis

Table 5.1 (*cont.*)

Growth factor	Source	Activities
IL-7	Marrow and thymus stromal cells	T and B cell lymphopoiesis
IL-8	Many cell types including macrophages	Chemo-attractant for T cells and neutrophils
IL-9	T cells	Thymopoietic and haematopoietic actions
IL-10	CD8+ B and T cells, activated TH_2 cells, macrophages	Inhibition of cellular immunity and cytokine synthesis; promotes B cell proliferation
IL-11	Stromal cells	Thrombopoietic, haematopoietic
IL-12	Macrophages, B cells	Promotion of cell-mediated immune reactions; INF-γ production & proliferation of NK cells
IL-13	TH_2 cells	Similar to IL-4
Interferons-α and β (INF-α and β)	Several somatic cell types, macrophages, neutrophils	Antiviral actions; NK cell, macrophage activation; activation of class I major histocompatibility complex (MHC) in somatic tissue
INF-γ	Activated NK, TH_1 cells	Similar to INF-α, -β; class II MHC activation; induction and activation of many immune cells; promotion of cell-mediated immunity
Nerve growth factor (NGF)	Nervous tissue	Promotion of neurite outgrowth and neural survival
Platelet-derived growth factor (PDGF)	Platelets	Induces several nuclear proto-oncogenes; promotes mesenchymal proliferation; cytoskeletal actions
Transforming growth factor-α (TGF-α)	Mainly carcinomas; some from epithelial tissues	Promotion of keratinocyte growth; together with TGF-β1 may transform normal cells
Transforming growth factor-β (TGF-β)	Diverse family, may run into hundreds of members, e.g. activins, inhibins	Proliferative in many different epithelial and mesenchymal cells. All have serine/threonine kinase activity; thus involved in intracellular signal cascades

[a] The list is not exhaustive.

Chapter 5 quiz

Answer T (true) or F (false)

1 GHRH releases GH from the posterior pituitary ☐
2 GH stimulates gluconeogenesis in muscle ☐
3 GH directly stimulates bone growth ☐
4 The growth hormone receptor activates intracellular kinases ☐
5 GH release is inhibited by pituitary somatostatin ☐
6 GH deficiency in children causes failure to grow ☐
7 GH deficiency is usually caused by hypothalamic–pituitary malfunction ☐
8 In children treatment of GH deficiency is with GH until adulthood ☐
9 GH excess is usually caused by bacterial infection ☐
10 GH excess causes gigantism in children ☐
11 Acromegaly results from excess GH in adults ☐
12 Acromegaly results in diabetes in all patients ☐
13 Acromegaly results in enlargement of the upper mandible ☐
14 GH excess is treated with dopamine agonists and surgery or radiation to remove tumours ☐

6 Human growth, growth disorders and treatments

Learning objectives
Normal human growth
Important causes of impaired growth and short
*   stature in children*
Symptoms and features of growth failure
Treatment of impaired growth
Treatment with growth hormone
Alternative therapy
Other potential uses of growth hormone

Learning objectives

- Appreciate what normal human growth and attainment of final height depend on
- Be able to list important causes of impaired growth and short stature in children
- Know the symptoms and features of growth failure
- Know the three main points about the approach to treatment of growth failure
- Be aware of the methods for monitoring growth during treatment

Normal human growth

Normal human growth and final height attainment after birth depend on:

- adequate secretion of GH by a normally functioning hypothalamic–pituitary axis (*see* Figure 5.1)
- normally functioning target organs for GH and other necessary growth factors (*see* below)
- normally functioning thyroid gland, especially during the early postnatal period
- normal sex hormone secretion during the pubertal growth spurt
- adequate nutrition, hygiene, absence of chronic disease
- genetic factors
- possibly an abuse-free home (*see* also below).

Important causes of impaired growth and short stature in children

- GH deficiency caused by congenital midline structural abnormalities of the hypothalamic–pituitary axis caused by birth trauma, perinatal CNS infection, autoimmune hypophysitis or hypothalamic or pituitary tumours
- Thyroid deficiency
- Prolonged glucocorticoid treatment during childhood
- Failure of normal pubertal sex hormone production and release
- Impaired release of GH and impaired function of other growth factors and receptors, especially IGF-1, due to poverty with poor nutrition and lack of hygiene, and possibly secondary cigarette smoke inhalation, drug abuse and alcohol
- Chronic diseases, especially those which impair food absorption, e.g. inflammatory bowel disease and coeliac disease
- Continual child abuse in an abnormal psychosocial home environment
- Idiopathic (unknown cause)

Symptoms and features of growth failure

- Height less than the third percentile
- Growth velocity less than 6 cm per year
- Immature facial appearance and abdominal obesity due to reduced lipolytic effects of GH
- Prominent forehead through deficient GH action on skeleton
- Reduced muscle mass
- High-pitched, immature voice

Treatment of impaired growth

Appropriate treatment depends on the correct diagnosis of impaired growth, and GH should be administered, if appropriate, as soon as possible, when normal growth rates will be established and maintained with continued treatment with GH until the child is fully grown.

Approach to treatment

- Identification of cause
- Institution of appropriate treatment, usually with recombinant GH as soon as possible
- Determination of growth velocity in comparison with standard growth charts and with the parental heights if these are within normal ranges

Treatment with growth hormone

- Treatment of GH-deficient children with recombinant (and therefore pathogen-free), natural-sequence GH at a dose-range, for younger children, of 0.18–0.3 mg/kg/week, administered once daily 6–7 times weekly until epiphyseal closure. Healthy thyroid function and adequate nutrition are necessary as well for treatment to succeed.
- Older children may require higher doses as advised by the clinician.
- Problems with treatment include:
    - (rarely) antibody development to GH
    - (rarely)development in younger and thinner children of slipped capital femoral epiphyses
    - symptoms of acromegaly (*see* p. 37) may develop with excessive use of GH.

Alternative therapy

- Use of recombinant derived IGF-1 in GH-resistant patients, e.g. Laron dwarfs, who cannot synthesise IGF-1
- Monitoring during treatment is essential by:
    - monitoring growth rate
    - regular assessment of bone age advancement
    - measurement of serum IGF-I and IGF-binding protein (IGFBP-3); (both should rise if treatment is successful)
    - measurement of serum bone alkaline phosphatase and urinary galactosyl-hydroxylysine, hydroxyproline and deoxypyridinolone

Other potential uses of growth hormone

- Promotion of wound healing rates
- Possible use in adults who suffered childhood deficiencies of GH

Chapter 6 quiz

Answer T (true) or F (false)

A   Normal growth and final height attainment depend on:
- Normally functioning gonads in early childhood
- Adequate secretion of growth hormone
- Normal thyroid function in the early postnatal period
- Adequate secretion of IGF-1 during the period of growth
- Genetic factors

B   Impaired growth may be due to:
- Insufficient intellectual stimulation during early childhood
- Chronic diseases which impair food absorption
- Prolonged treatment with glucocorticoids during childhood
- Poor nutrition during growth
- Thyroid over-activity during growth

C   Symptoms and features of growth failure include:
- Hirsutism
- Growth velocity less than 6 cm per year
- Reduced muscle mass
- Skeletal abnormalities caused by GH deficiency
- High-pitched voice
- Height less than the second percentile

D   Treatment of impaired growth involves:
- Diagnosis of cause
- Treatment with recombinant sex hormones
- Treatment with recombinant GH
- Regular comparison with standard growth curves
- Treatment until epiphyseal closure

E   Monitoring during treatment involves:
- Regular IQ tests
- Measurement of serum IGF-1 and IGFBP-3
- Measurement of plasma haemoglobin
- Measurement of serum bone alkaline phosphatase
- Regular assessment of bone age advancement

7 Steroidogenesis

Learning objectives
Definitions
Chemical structures of major steroid hormones
Major organs of steroid hormone biosynthesis
Major cellular sites of steroidogenesis
Control of steroidogenesis
Pathways of steroidogenesis
Summary of steroidogenic enzyme deficiencies

Learning objectives

- Know the major classes of steroid hormones and their main actions
- Be able to list the major steroid-producing tissues and the steroid hormones they produce
- Know the cellular sites of steroid hormone synthesis
- Have a basic knowledge of the control of steroidogenesis in the major steroid-producing tissues and organs
- Read through and have some knowledge of the various steroidogenic enzyme deficiencies and their consequences

Definitions

- *Steroidogenesis*: biosynthesis of the steroids (*see* below)
- *Steroid*: a chemical possessing the steroid nucleus, which is the cyclopentanoperhydrophenanthrene nucleus (*see* Figure 7.1)

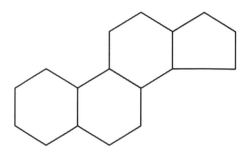

Figure 7.1 Cyclopentanoperhydrophenanthrene nucleus.

- *Steroid hormone*: hormone containing the steroid nucleus; examples of classes are:
  - *androgens*: responsible for male attributes, e.g. *testosterone*
  - *estrogens*: responsible for female attributes, e.g. *estradiol*
  - *progestogens* (progestins): necessary for the success of fertilisation and implantation and for normal maintenance of pregnancy, principally *progesterone*
  - *corticosteroids*: steroids synthesised in the adrenal cortex; two main types are synthesised: *glucocorticoids*: responsible for (i) a normal response to stress; (ii) correct utilisation of carbohydrates, fats and proteins, e.g. *cortisol*; and *mineralocorticoids*: necessary for salt, especially NaCl, and water balance, e.g. *aldosterone*

Note: be careful not to confuse the physiological actions of corticosteroids with the pharmacological actions of synthetic glucocorticoids, e.g. prednisolone.

Chemical structures of major steroid hormones

The structures of five major steroid hormones are shown in Figures 7.2 to 7.6 below.

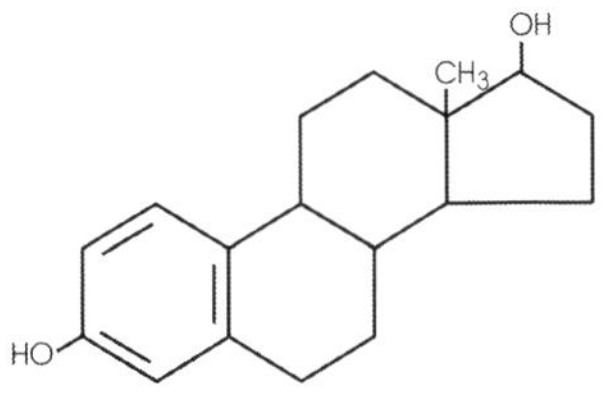

Figure 7.2 Estradiol.

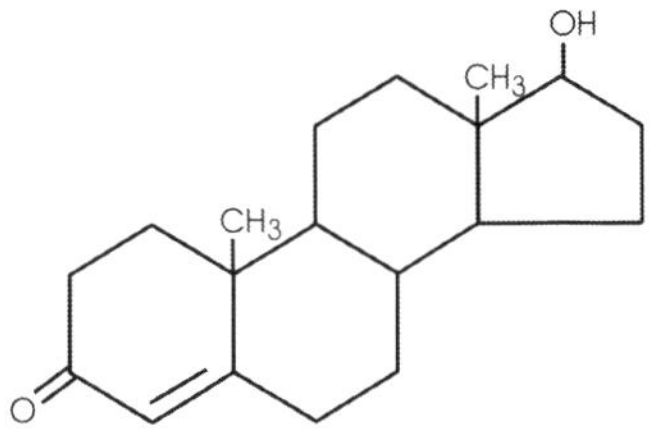

Figure 7.3 Testosterone.

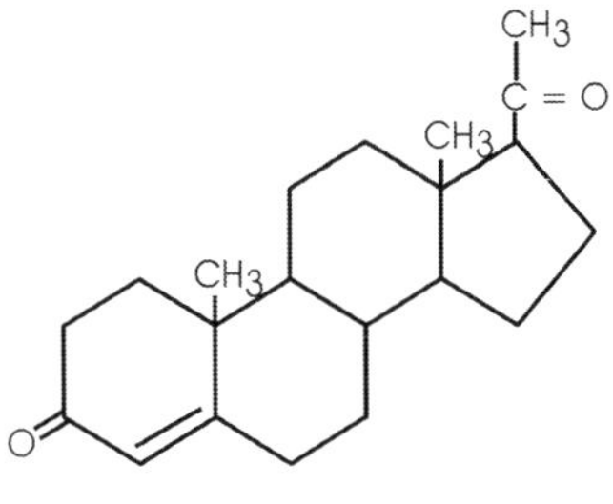

Figure 7.4 Progesterone.

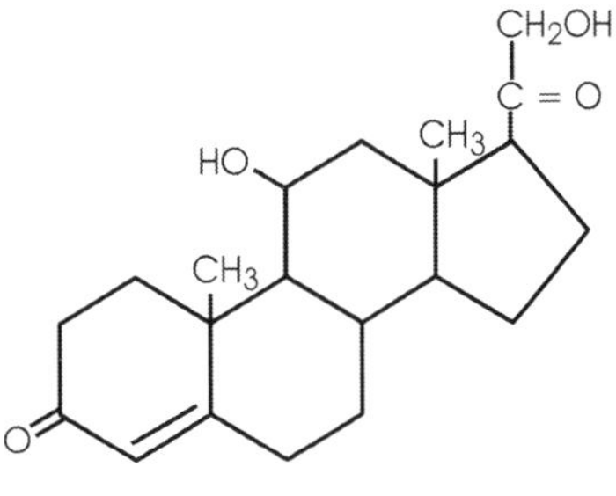

Figure 7.5 Cortisol.

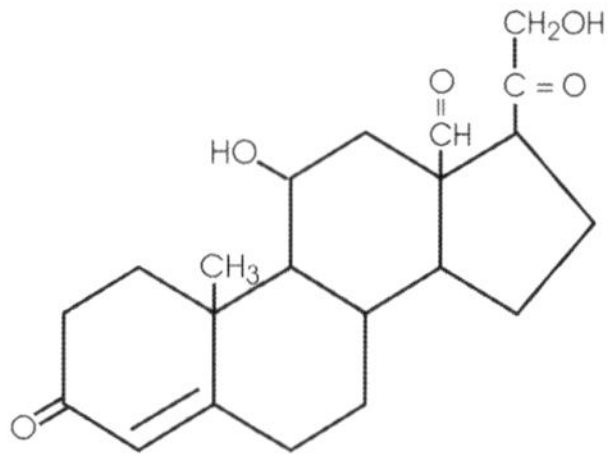

Figure 7.6 Aldosterone.

Major organs of steroid hormone biosynthesis

- *Androgens*: testis; adrenal cortex (*see* Figures 7.7 and 7.8; normally less important for sexual function[1])
- *Estrogens*: ovary (*see* Figure 7.8); adrenal cortex (normally less important for sexual function[2])
- *Glucocorticoids*: adrenal cortex
- *Mineralocorticoids*: adrenal cortex

Major cellular sites of steroidogenesis

- *Androgens*: Leydig (interstitial) cells of the testis; zona fasciculata and reticularis of adrenal cortex
- *Estrogens*: granulosa cells of the ovary; small amounts in the adrenal zona fasciculata and reticularis
- *Progesterone*: Mainly the corpus luteum and placenta; small amounts in the adrenal cortex
- *Cortisol*: mainly the adrenal zona fasciculata
- *Aldosterone*: adrenal zona glomerulosa (*see* note below) and outermost layers of the zona fasciculata

---

Note: this means that the zona glomerulosa is the only adrenal zone absolutely essential for life, since unregulated salt and water loss is potentially fatal.

---

[1] On their own androgens are insufficient to maintain normal male function.
[2] On their own estrogens are insufficient to maintain normal female function.

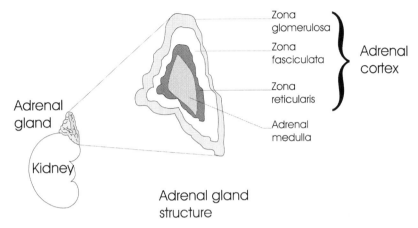

Figure 7.7 Adrenal gland structure.

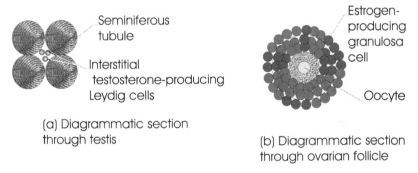

Figure 7.8 Steroid-producing cells in the testis and ovary. Diagrammatic sections through (a) the testis; (b) the ovarian follicle.

Control of steroidogenesis

- *Rate-limiting step in steroidogenesis*: action of steroidogenic acute regulatory protein (StAR) on transport of cholesterol from the outer to the inner mitochondrial membrane (*see* Figure 7.9)
- *Adrenal cortex*: action of ACTH on adrenal cortical cells
- *Testis*: action of LH on testicular Leydig (interstitial) cell
- *Ovary*: action of LH on ovarian granulosa cell
- *Placenta*: action of HCG, which stimulates progesterone production

Pathways of steroidogenesis

A general overview of steroidogenesis is shown in Figure 7.9.

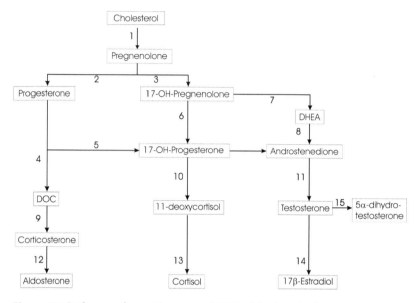

Figure 7.9 Pathways of steroidogenesis. DHEA, dehydroepiandrosterone; enzyme reactions are as follows:

1 cholesterol 20, 22 side chain cleavage (CYP11A1, modern nomenclature)
2 3β-hydroxysteroid dehydrogenase (3-β-HSD)
3 17α-hydroxylase (CYP17)
4 21α-hydroxylase (CYP21A2)
5 17α-hydroxylase
6 3β-hydroxysteroid dehydrogenase
7 17α-hydroxylase/17,20 lyase (CYP17)
8 3β-hydroxysteroid dehydrogenase
9 11β-hydroxylase (CYP11B1)
10 21α-hydroxylase
11 17β-hydroxysteroid dehydrogenase
12 aldosterone synthase (CYP11B2)
13 11β-hydroxylase
14 P450 aromatase (CYP19)
15 5α-reductase.

Summary of steroidogenic enzyme deficiencies

Aetiology: these are inherited autosomal recessive deficiencies of enzymes of steroidogenesis, resulting mainly in deficiencies of cortisol and aldosterone, which allow the build-up of intermediates that are shunted into other pathways, notably into androgen-producing pathways (*see* Table 7.1). The overall results are often:

- over-stimulation of ACTH release, which causes hyperplasia of the adrenal cortex and overproduction of androgens. This results in virilisation
- in some cases (*see* below) normal development of gonads and secondary sex glands is impaired, together with puberty failure
- hypertension due to excess release of DOC.

Table 7.1 Enzyme deficiencies, their consequences and treatment

Enzyme deficiency	Consequences	Treatment
11β-hydroxylase (CYP11B1)	Adrenal hyperplasia; hypertension, possibly due to raised 11-DOC; cortisol lack; virilisation due to excess androgen production	Restore physiological levels of glucocorticoids
17α-hydroxylase (CYP17)	Adrenal hyperplasia; at puberty, hypogonadism, hypertension and hypokalaemia; in some cases abnormal gonadal and secondary sex gland development	Glucocorticoids to suppress ACTH; replacement with gonadal sex steroids
3β-hydroxysteroid dehydrogenase (rare)	Adrenal hyperplasia; all steroid hormone classes reduced; failure of normal gonadal and sexual development	Steroid replacement and suppression of excess adrenal dehydroepiandrosterone (DHEA) and pituitary ACTH release
21α-hydroxylase (CYP21A2; the most common)	Adrenal hyperplasia; androgen excess and virilisation; infertility in women	Suppression of ACTH with glucocorticoid therapy; mineralocorticoid replacement; inhibition of excess androgenisation; reconstructive surgery if necessary
StAR deficiency (rarest form of deficiency; congenital lipoid hyperplasia)	All adrenal steroids deficient; fatal in ∼ two-thirds of all patients reported	Glucocorticoid and mineralocorticoid replacement

Chapter 7 quiz

Answer T (true) or F (false)

1 Androgens are hormones responsible for the male attributes ☐
2 Estrogens are hormones responsible for female attributes ☐
3 Progesterone is not necessary for implantation ☐
4 Corticosteroids are synthesised in the adrenal medulla ☐
5 Aldosterone is synthesised mainly in the zona fasciculata ☐
6 HCG stimulates progesterone production by the feto-placental unit ☐
7 17α-hydroxylase converts pregnenolone to 17α-hydroxypregnenolone ☐
8 11β-hydroxylase converts 17α-hydroxyprogesterone to cortisol ☐
9 Testosterone can be converted to estradiol ☐
10 Cortisol is converted directly to aldosterone in the zona glomerulosa ☐
11 Over-stimulation by ACTH causes adrenocortical hyperplasia ☐
12 Steroidogenic enzyme deficiencies can result in failure of puberty ☐
13 Over-stimulation by ACTH can result in hypertension ☐
14 11β-hydroxylase deficiency can result in virilisation ☐
15 StAR deficiency is the commonest steroidogenic enzyme deficiency ☐

8 Sexual differentiation and pathophysiology

Learning objectives
Classification of sexual differentiation
Hormonal determinants of normal reproductive
system development and secondary sexual
characteristics
Pathophysiology of human sexual differentiation

Learning objectives

- Understand the difference between genetic and gonadal sex
- Be aware of the hormonal determinants of sexual development and be able to give some examples of that role
- Be acquainted with the examples given here of human differentiation pathophysiology

Classification of sexual differentiation

- *Genetic sex* is determined by the sex chromosomes. XX is female and XY is male. Genetic sex is determined when male and female gametes fuse at conception. If the Y chromosome is absent, the female genitalia and female phenotype will develop.
- *Gonadal sex* refers to the presence of an ovary or testis, whose presence and proper function are required for sexual female and male reproductive competence respectively.

Terminology notes: *genotype* refers to the genetic constitution of the individual, e.g. XX or XY. *Phenotype* refers to the observable characteristics (secondary sexual characteristics) of the individual, resulting from the expression of the genes.

Consequence of Y chromosome possession

The Y chromosome possesses a gene called the *Sry* gene, which expresses the *Sry antigen*. The Sry antigen switches on genes responsible for development of the testes.

53

Hormonal determinants of normal reproductive system development and secondary sexual characteristics

- *Secondary sexual characteristics* determine the phenotype, e.g. female breast and external genitalia development, and male typical muscular configuration, hair distribution and external genitalia development, as well as development of male accessory sex organs (*see* Figure 8.1).
- *In the absence of a testis*, the female phenotype develops, together with the internal secondary sexual organs, i.e. the fallopian tube, uterus and part of the vagina, which are formed from the Müllerian (paramesonephric) ducts.
- *In the presence of a testis*, the testis produces a hormone, the Müllerian inhibiting hormone, called *anti-Müllerian hormone* (AMH), which causes

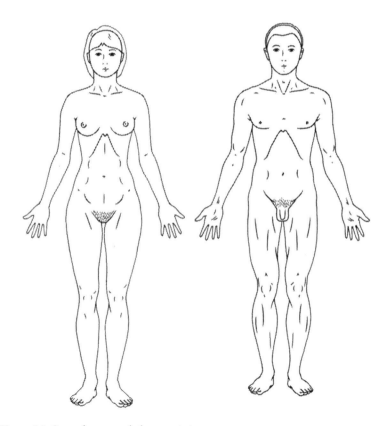

Figure 8.1 Secondary sexual characteristics.

the Müllerian ducts to atrophy. The testis also produces *testosterone*, which promotes the development of the *Wolffian ducts*, which will develop into the ductus deferens, epididymis and seminal vesicles.

Development of the external genitalia

In the presence of the Y chromosome and testosterone, the fetal scrotum and testes develop and the testes descend into the scrotum. In the absence of the Y chromosome the labia and clitoris will develop.

> *Note:* if neither the ovaries nor the testes develop, the Müllerian ducts will continue to develop, and the male Wolffian ducts will atrophy. Therefore neither male nor female gonads are necessary for female ductal differentiation and development.

Pathophysiology of human sexual differentiation[1]

- *Klinefelter's syndrome*: males have an extra X chromosome and may be 'classic' type (47XXY; the more usual), or 'mosaic' (46XY/47XXY). Other, rarer mosaics also occur. *Adult features* are infertility, gynaecomastia (breast development), tall stature, small testes and penis, azoospermia (complete absence of sperm), reduced circulating testosterone and gonadotrophins, reduced facial hair, reduced sexual function.
- *Gonadal dysgenesis – Turner syndrome* and variant forms: affected women possess only one X chromosome. *Adult features* are short stature, perhaps webbing of the skin of the neck or other developmental abnormalities; presence of external genitalia but absence of ovaries and therefore of menstruation; infertility.
- *Gonadal dysgenesis – 'male Turner syndrome'*: occurrence in some phenotypic males of webbed neck, short stature and undescended testes.
- *True hermaphroditism*: rare; the individual has both ovarian and testicular tissue in opposite or the same gonads. Karyotypes[2] are 46XX, 46XX/46XY or, rarely, 46XY, usually inheritance is autosomal recessive; at puberty both breast development and virilisation occur. Treatment, if decided upon, may be sex assignment, e.g. 46XX may dictate female assignment.
- *Pseudohermaphroditism*: congenitally determined abnormality when the male or female external genitalia resemble those of the opposite sex, e.g. inappropriate presence of androgens (due to, e.g. adrenal enzyme deficiencies) causes partial masculinisation of the clitoris and, if left untreated, male musculature and baldness.

[1] This is a highly condensed summary of a very complex pathology.
[2] Karyotype defines the chromosome set in terms of chromosome type and number.

Note: *congenital adrenal hyperplasia* (CAH): most cases of ambiguous external genitalia and of female pseudohermaphroditism occur because of mutations in one or more steroidogenic enzymes CYP11A1, CYP17, CYP21, HSD3B2 or in StAR (*see* also above).

Chapter 8 quiz

Answer T (true) or F (false)

A Genetic sex:
- Is determined by the sex chromosomes
- Determines the secondary sexual characteristics
- Defines the genotype

B The phenotype refers to:
- The genetic constitution of the individual
- The observable secondary sexual characteristics

C The Sry antigen:
- Is on the X chromosome
- Switches on genes responsible for testis development

D Secondary sexual characteristics include:
- The ovary
- Muscular configuration
- Hair distribution
- Accessory sex organs
- External genitalia

E In the absence of a testis:
- The male phenotype still develops
- The female internal secondary sex organs develop

F The female Müllerian ducts give rise to:
- The ovary
- The Wolffian ducts
- The fallopian tubes, uterus and part of the vagina

G In the presence of a testis:
- The Müllerian ducts atrophy
- The Wolffian ducts atrophy
- Testosterone is produced
- The ductus deferens, epididymis and seminal vesicles develop

H In the absence of both ovary and testis:
- The Wolffian ducts develop
- The Müllerian ducts continue to develop

I Klinefelter's syndrome:
- Occurs when males have an extra Y chromosome
- Is characterised by infertility and gynaecomastia

- Is characterised by enlarged testis and penis ☐
- Causes reduced testosterone and sperm production ☐

J Turner's syndrome:
- Is a genetic defect when women possess an extra X chromosome ☐
- Results in:
  - absence of external genitalia ☐
  - absence of ovaries ☐
  - webbing of the neck ☐
  - short stature ☐
  - infertility ☐

K Individuals with true hermaphroditism:
- Possess both ovarian and testicular tissue ☐
- Feature breast development and virilisation ☐
- May be treated by sex assignment, depending on chromosomal karyotype ☐

L Congenital adrenal hyperplasia:
- Is the most common cause of ambiguous external genitalia ☐
- Occurs due to the absence of the testis ☐

9 Puberty

Learning objectives
What is puberty?
Features of puberty
Disorders of puberty

Learning objectives

- Be able to describe the features of puberty in males and females
- Learn the symptoms and treatments of delayed puberty
- Appreciate the distinction between true precocious puberty and pseudo-precocious puberty
- Be able to list the symptoms and treatment of precocious puberty

What is puberty?

Puberty is a developmental milestone when the reproductive organs become functional.

Features of puberty (see Figure 9.1)

- Growth spurt
- Maturation of the hypothalamo–pituitary axis, resulting in increase in gonadal steroidal and growth hormone secretion, possibly due to reduced sensitivity of the central nervous system (CNS) to negative feedback effects of testosterone and estrogens, resulting in:
  - growth of accessory and external sex organs in male and female
  - poorly understood changes in mood and behaviour

Male puberty

Onset of spermatogenesis and increased androgen activity of testosterone and its metabolite 5α-dihydrotestosterone (DHT), which causes:

- penis, scrotum and testis enlargement
- penis and scrotum pigmentation
- prostate, epididymis and seminal vesicle growth
- male pattern of hair distribution
- linear growth acceleration with growth of connective tissue and muscle
- enlargement of larynx and thickening of vocal cords
- fall in plasma HDL

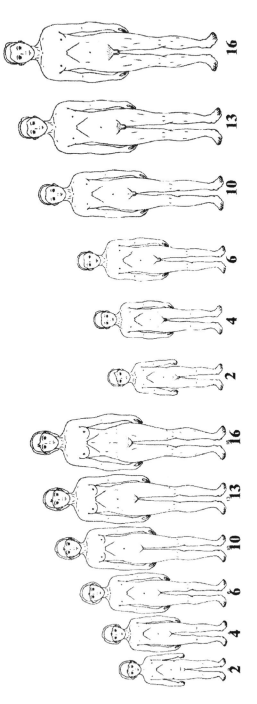

Figure 9.1 Human growth to puberty. Adapted from Cull P (ed). *The Sourcebook of Medical Illustration.* Carnforth: The Parthenon Publishing Group, 1989.

- increase in the haematocrit[1]
- behavioural and psychological changes associated with increased libido.[2]

Female puberty

- onset of adrenal androgen secretion (adrenarche)
- increased pituitary sensitivity to GnRH
- reduced sensitivity of the CNS to negative feedback effects of gonadal steroids
- increased production and secretion of estrogens by the ovarian follicle and the onset of ovulatory menstrual cycles
- development of breasts, female pattern of fat deposition and distribution of body hair

> *Note:* there is a critical minimum body weight of about 48–50 kg, below which menstrual cycles do not occur; this explains why extreme dieting, malnutrition and heavy involvement in sport may stop menstrual cycles.

Disorders of puberty[3]

Sexual infantilism and delayed puberty

- *Constitutional delayed puberty:* delay not associated with any pathological condition; may be familial and does not affect normal reproductive activity after puberty has occurred
- Sexual infantilism may occur due to:
  - failure of gonadotrophin secretion caused by CNS or pituitary tumours
  - congenital deficiency of GnRH production (Kallman's syndrome)
  - childhood obesity linked to hyperphagia (dietary excess)
  - other endocrine problems, e.g. poorly controlled diabetes mellitus, Cushing's disease
  - anorexia nervosa (mainly girls)
  - iatrogenic aetiology – caused by treatment for other disorders, e.g. irradiation; cytotoxic drug therapy
  - head trauma

---

[1] Haematocrit is the volume of red cells as a fraction of total blood volume; also called the packed cell volume.
[2] Libido: sexual drive.
[3] This list is not exhaustive.

Treatment of sexual infantilism and delayed puberty
Constitutional delays are generally not treated.

Strategies for treatment
- Identification and correction (or removal, if possible) of lesion
- Induction of normal hormonal blood levels to promote development of the gonads, accessory sex organs and secondary sexual characteristics
- Follow-up monitoring of pubertal changes and, if necessary, repeat treatment
- If necessary, permanent hormonal replacement regimes
- Psychosocial support and counselling

Hormonal substitution therapy[4]
- *Girls*:
  - treatment with synthetic oral estrogen e.g. ethinylestradiol daily for 4–6 months or until 'breakthrough' bleeding occurs, followed by cyclic regimes of treatment to mimic normal estrogen–progesterone pattern of cyclic release
  - induction of ovulation, if necessary, with e.g. pulsatile GnRH (*see* p. 61)
- *Boys*:
  - at 13 years or when diagnosed, testosterone enanthate or other long-active testosterone ester (usually administered intramuscular (IM)) monthly for 6–12 months, after which dose and dose frequency are gradually increased to approximate to normal male age-related increases in testosterone secretion
  - for induction of fertility, males may be treated with e.g. pulsatile GnRH

Precocious puberty
True precocious puberty (gonadotrophin-dependent puberty)
True precocious puberty is caused by inappropriate secretion of pituitary gonadotrophins, usually at 8–9 years of age.

- The cause may be idiopathic.[5]
- In some cases MRI and CT scans have shown abnormal brain development when ectopic[6] GnRH-secreting neurones have been localised e.g. in brain tumours.
- It may occur in acquired hypothyroidism.

---

[4] Examples are given, but different conditions may require alternative strategies.
[5] Cause unknown.
[6] Here this means cells or tissues misplaced, usually through congenital abnormalities.

> *Reminder.* GnRH stimulates the release of pituitary gonadotrophins LH and FSH.

Pseudoprecocious puberty

Pseudoprecocious puberty is caused by inappropriate release of *pituitary* LH or FSH. There are several types, all of which result in secretion of sex hormones or gonadotrophins:

- adrenal tumours or congenital conditions, e.g. congenital adrenal hyperplasia (CAH)
- ectopic tissues which secrete gonadotrophins
- gonadal tumours, e.g. ovarian cysts or tumours of testicular Leydig cells, which produce testosterone
- the McCune–Albright syndrome, more prevalent in girls, is usually due to ovarian cysts and may occur as early as three years of age.

Symptoms and consequences of precocious puberty

- Breast enlargement
- Growth of pubic and axillary (underarm) hair
- Growth of external genitalia
- In boys, acne, erections and nocturnal ejaculation
- Weight gain and abnormal tallness for their age, although they experience premature epiphysial closure and cessation of height gain

Treatment of precocious puberty

Primary aims

- Block the secretion and actions of inappropriately released hormones and mediators
- Remove sources of these secretions if possible

Treatments

- Removal of tumours, if possible
- Chemical intervention:
  - GnRH analogues, e.g. buserelin to suppress sex hormone production, and GH to improve height attainment potential
  - sex hormone receptor blocking drugs, e.g. the anti-androgen cyproterone
  - treatment with glucocorticoids for CAH

Chapter 9 quiz

Answer T (true) or F (false)

1 Adrenarche is cessation of adrenal androgen production in girls ☐

2 True precocious puberty is caused by inappropriate gonadotrophin release from the pituitary gland ☐

3 Pseudoprecocious puberty is caused by ectopic secretion of sex hormones or gonadotrophins ☐

A Male puberty is characterised by:
- Enlargement of the larynx and vocal cord thickening ☐
- Penis and scrotum pigmentation ☐
- Growth of accessory sex organs ☐
- Rise in plasma HDL ☐
- Acceleration of linear growth ☐
- Onset of spermatogenesis ☐
- Increased androgen activity ☐

B Female puberty is characterised by:
- Increased CNS sensitivity to negative feedback by estrogen ☐
- Increased pituitary sensitivity to hypothalamic GnRH ☐
- Increased production and secretion of estrogen by the ovarian corpus luteum ☐
- Breast development and a female pattern of fat deposition ☐

C Sexual infantilism may be due to:
- Anorexia nervosa ☐
- Congenital overproduction of GnRH ☐
- CNS or pituitary tumours ☐
- Childhood obesity ☐
- Other endocrine problems e.g. Cushing's disease ☐
- Drug treatments e.g. use of cytotoxic drugs ☐

D Treatment of sexual infantilism and delayed puberty involves:
- Identification of a possible lesion, e.g. tumour ☐
- Hormonal replacement to mimic the normal situation ☐
- Follow-up monitoring of pubertal changes and more treatment if necessary ☐
- Permanent hormonal regime establishment if needed ☐

E Hormonal therapy for girls may involve:
- Treatment with a GnRH antagonist ☐
- Treatment with synthetic oral estrogens to induce 'breakthrough' bleeding ☐
- Establishment of estrogen–progestogen regimes to mimic cyclic hormonal release ☐

F   Hormonal therapy for boys may involve:
- Treatment with implants of GnRH
- Long-acting testosterone analogues

10 Female sex organs and the menstrual cycle

Learning objectives
Anatomical location of female sex organs
The ovary
Components of the female reproductive tract
A definition of the menstrual cycle
Major hormones of the menstrual cycle
Follicular development
Ovarian synthesis of estradiol
Phases of the menstrual cycle
Disorders of the menstrual cycle

Learning objectives

- Be able to sketch quickly the layout of the ovary and the rest of the reproductive tract
- Know the essential functions of the components of the reproductive tract
- Be able to list the major female sex hormones, the four stages of follicular development and the phases of the menstrual cycle
- Have an awareness of menstrual cycle disorders

Anatomical location of female sex organs

The female sex organs are located in the lower abdomen (*see* Figure 10.1).

The ovary

The ovary is the female gonad[1]:

- **Anatomical location:** two ovaries bilaterally in the lower abdomen
- **Structure** (*see* Figure 10.2): contains an outer *cortex* where follicles mainly occur and an inner *medulla* containing nerves and blood vessels
- **Functions:** mainly synthesis of female sex steroids, principally estradiol, and production of the ovum by the follicles

---

[1] The gonads are the organs in which the gametes (ovum and spermatozoa) are made. The male gonad is the testis.

66

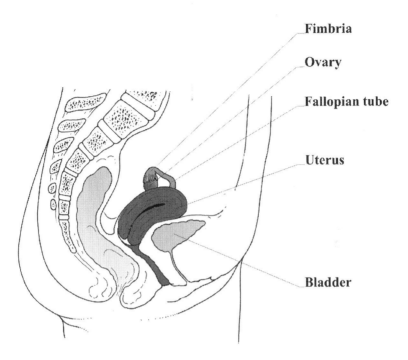

Figure 10.1 Sagittal section showing the female reproductive organs (only one ovary shown).

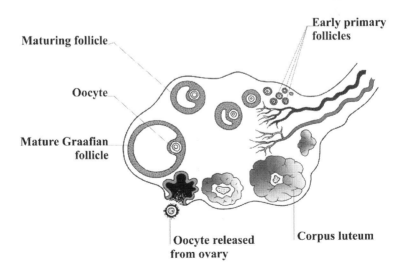

Figure 10.2 Section through the ovary.

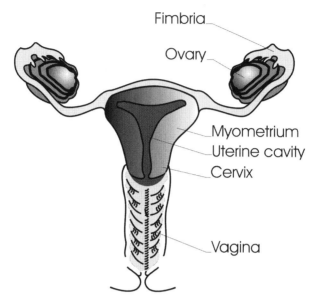

Figure 10.3 The female reproductive tract.

Components of the female reproductive tract (see Figure 10.3)

- *Fallopian tubes*: bilateral pair of tubes that conduct ova (eggs) released from the ovary (*see* below) to the uterus
- *Fimbria*: fringe-like processes at the ovarian end of the fallopian tubes, which catch the free-floating ovum
- *Uterus* (womb): part of reproductive tract with an inner *endometrium* specialised for implantation of the fertilized ovum, and outer *myometrium* (smooth muscle) for expulsion of the fully developed fetus at birth
- *Cervix*: neck-like part of the uterus, projecting into the:
- *Vagina*: muscular tube lined with a mucous membrane, linking the uterus with the external environment

A definition of the menstrual cycle

The menstrual cycle is a periodic sequence of endocrine-driven events in non-pregnant, sexually mature women, directed towards:

- the production and release into the reproductive canal of a fertilisable egg cell or ovum
- creation of an endometrium able to effect the successful implantation of a fertilised egg.

Major hormones of the menstrual cycle

- Estradiol
- Progesterone
- LH
- FSH

Note: many other hormones and chemical mediators are involved in the menstrual cycle.

Follicular development

There are four main stages of follicular development:

1 the primordial follicle
2 early and late primary follicles
3 secondary follicles
4 mature (Graafian) follicles.

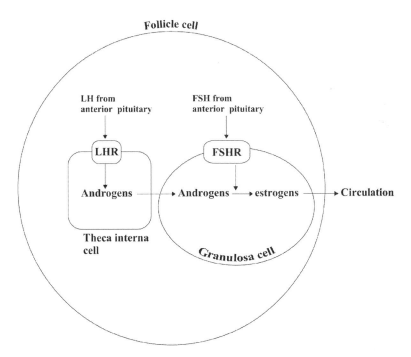

Figure 10.4 Biosynthesis of estrogens in the ovary. LHR, LH receptor; FSHR, FSH receptor.

Ovarian synthesis of estradiol (*see* Figure 10.4)

During the follicular phase of the menstrual cycle, FSH causes follicular growth and stimulates conversion of ovarian androgens to estrogens, i.e. estradiol and estrone.

Phases of the menstrual cycle

Phases of the menstrual cycle are shown in Table 10.1 (*see* also Figure 10.5).

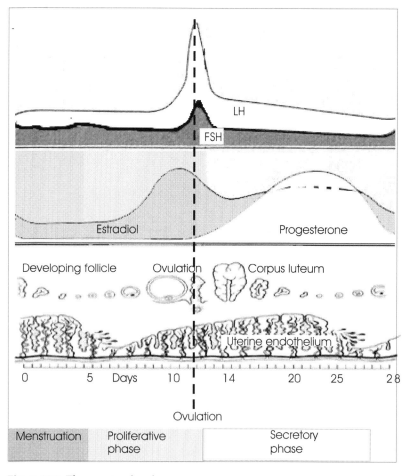

Figure 10.5 The menstrual cycle.

Table 10.1 Phases of the menstrual cycle (*see* also Figure 10.5)

Event	Duration[a]	Plasma hormonal activity
1 Menses	4–5 days	LH, FSH low
2 Proliferative follicular phase	8–11 days	Estradiol rises to peak ±24 h before ovulation; progesterone low
3 Ovulation	24 hours	Estradiol causes LH, FSH surges from the pituitary; estradiol is decreasing; progesterone low
4 Secretory luteal phase	13–15 days	Estradiol declines to mid-luteal plateau; progesterone rises; LH, FSH levels decline

[a] There are very many individual variations.

Notes:

- In the granulosa cell, estradiol stimulates production of the hormone *inhibin*, which is released into the circulation and, during the proliferative phase, has a negative feedback effect on FSH release.
- Estrogens stimulate progesterone receptor synthesis, thus 'priming' the tissues for progesterone action.

Disorders of the menstrual cycle

- *Amenorrhoea*: absence or cessation of menstrual periods:
  - *primary*: failure to appear at puberty
  - *secondary*: periods stop occurring
- *Dysmenorrhoea*: painful menstruation:
  - *primary* (spasmodic): usually begins with first period
  - *secondary* (congestive): affects mainly older women; causes include an intrauterine device (IUD), uterine fibroids, pelvic inflammatory disease
- *Menorrhagia* (epimenorrhagia): abnormally heavy bleeding during menstruation
- *Metrorrhagia*: bleeding from the uterus at times different from normally expected menstruation; this should always be investigated as it may be a symptom of a serious condition
- *Premenstrual syndrome* (PMS; also called premenstrual tension (PMT)): emotional disturbances which may include irritability, nervousness, depression, headache; symptoms usually disappear at the onset of menstruation

Chapter 10 quiz

Answer T (true) or F (false)

1 The ovarian functions are mainly sex hormone and ovum production ☐

2 Follicles develop in the cortex of the ovary ☐

3 The fertilised egg is implanted in the uterine myometrium ☐

4 The fimbria conduct eggs to the uterus ☐

5 Menses occurs just before menstrual flow ☐

6 The mature follicle is called a Graafian follicle ☐

7 FSH promotes conversion of androgens to estrogens in the ovary ☐

8 FSH inhibits follicular growth ☐

9 The follicular (proliferative) phase lasts about 8–11 days ☐

10 Ovulation lasts about 1 hour ☐

11 The luteal (secretory) phase lasts about 13–15 days ☐

12 Estradiol stimulates progesterone receptor synthesis ☐

13 Estrogen stimulates inhibin secretion in the ovarian granulosa cell ☐

14 Inhibin inhibits pituitary secretion of FSH ☐

15 Amenorrhoea is abnormally frequent menstrual periods ☐

16 Dysmenorrhoea is painful menstruation ☐

17 Secondary dysmenorrhoea affects mainly younger women ☐

18 Menorrhagia is abnormally heavy bleeding during menstruation ☐

19 Metrorrhagia is unexpected bleeding from the vagina outside normally expected periods and should always be investigated ☐

11 Female sex hormones and their receptors

Learning objectives
Estradiol
Estrone and estriol
Progesterone

Learning objectives

- Be familiar with the concept of A ring aromatisation in the biosynthesis of estrogens
- Be able to list the principal physiological actions of estradiol
- Appreciate the influence of estradiol absence at menopause
- Be able to draw the given mechanism of action of estradiol (*see* Figure 11.1)
- Know what is meant by SERMs and be able to give examples and some important uses
- Know some important therapeutic uses of estrogens
- Be able to discuss briefly the known and suspected impact of estrogens on diseases, notably breast cancer and cardiovascular disease
- Be able to list the physiological actions of progesterone, and have knowledge of some important therapeutic uses of synthetic progestogens

Female sex steroid hormones are:

- Estradiol
- Estrone
- Estriol
- Progesterone

Estradiol

Biosynthesis

See p. 50.

Physiological actions of estradiol

Puberty

- Stimulation of the endometrium, myometrium, vaginal growth and breast stroma

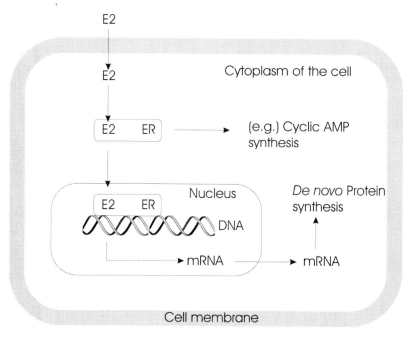

Figure 11.1 Genomic and extragenomic action of estrogen receptors. ER, estrogen receptor; E2, estradiol.

- Female pattern of fat deposition
- Epiphyseal closure

Adult female
- Maintenance of female secondary characteristics (*see* Figure 8.1)
- Maintenance of the menstrual cycle
- Promotion of progesterone receptor synthesis
- Female sexual behaviour?

Pregnancy
- Ductal proliferation in the breasts
- Fluid retention enhanced
- Blood flow increase through the uterus
- Hypertrophy of uterine myometrium
- Promotion of progesterone receptor synthesis
- Stimulation of oxytocin receptor synthesis in uterine myometrium

Metabolic actions
- Increases plasma HDL and decreases plasma LDL
- Decreases total plasma cholesterol
- Stimulates production of coagulation factors II, VII, IX and X
- Decreases platelet aggregation
- Stimulates production in the liver of plasma SHBG and thyroxin-binding globulin
- Inhibits bone resorption
- Decreases bowel motility

Menopause
Estrogen's actions are manifested through their cessation at menopause:

- vasomotor instability, e.g. sweating, hot flushes
- increased rate of bone resorption
- dryness of the vagina due to decreased secretions
- mood and behavioural changes due to estrogen lack?

Mechanisms of action of estradiol (see Figure 11.1)

The actions of estradiol on the cell are mediated by specific estrogen receptors. There are two main subtypes encoded by different genes:

- ER-alpha (ERα)
- ER-beta (ERβ).

Both subtypes express the actions of estradiol through:

- *genomic mechanisms*: i.e. they alter gene expression and protein synthesis (actions apparent within hours)
- *non-genomic actions*: e.g. activation of protein kinases in the cytoplasm (actions apparent within seconds or minutes).

Drugs developed to counteract or modify actions of estrogens

Selective estrogen receptor modulators (SERMs)
These are synthetic compounds which compete with endogenous[1] estradiol for its receptor sites and they block or modulate the actions of the hormone. Examples are:

- raloxifene
- tamoxifen.

---

[1] Endogenous means produced in the body as opposed to exogenous, which means originating outside the body.

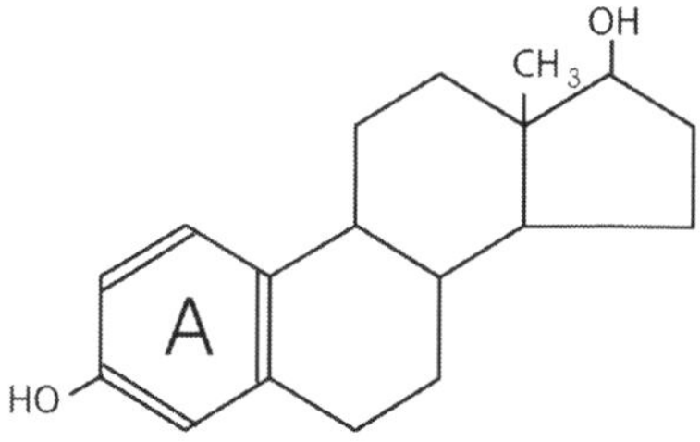

Estradiol

Figure 11.2 The A ring of estradiol.

Aromatase inhibitors

These drugs inhibit the aromatase enzyme system which catalyses the formation of the aromatic A ring of the estrogens (*see* Figure 11.2).

Examples are:

- anastrozole
- exemestane
- letrozole

Examples of synthetic estrogens

- Diethylstilbestrol (mainly of historical interest now)
- Ethinylestradiol
- Estradiol esters:
  - estradiol cypionate
  - estradiol valerate
- Mestranol

Therapeutic uses of estrogens

- Oral contraceptives (*see* p. 90)
- Hormone replacement therapy (HRT)
- Replacement therapy in primary hypogonadism
- Hirsutism and amenorrhoea caused by over-secretion of androgens
- Suppression of excessive bleeding caused by endometrial hyperplasia

Estrogens and disease

Medical problems with evidence of estradiol involvement:

- cancer
- post-menopausal osteoporosis
- cardiovascular disease
- neurodegenerative disease

Estrogens and cancer
- *Breast cancer*: estradiol may initiate and exacerbate breast cancer. Tumour biopsies may stain positive or negative for estrogen receptors, and SERMs and aromatase inhibitors are indicated for those that stain positive.
- *Prostate cancer* (*see* also p. 77): diethylstilbestrol, a synthetic estrogen, was extensively used in the past to treat prostate cancer, since there is some evidence that estrogens are protective.

Estrogens and postmenopausal osteoporosis
Estrogen deficiency is associated with increased bone resorption and there is much evidence that HRT (*see* also p. 101) reduces the incidence of fractures in postmenopausal women.

Estrogens and cardiovascular diseases
There is a significant increase in the incidence of cardiovascular diseases after menopause, and this may be due, in part, to the loss of estrogens, which are known to lower plasma LDL and increase HDL, although genetic factors may also be important.

Estrogens and neurodegenerative disease
There is evidence that endogenous estrogens protect against neurodegenerative disease through:

- decreasing the dangers of stroke
- protecting neurones against cell death, although this aspect is still very tentative, albeit interesting.

Estrone and estriol
- *Estrone* is a relatively weak metabolite of estradiol, produced in the liver, gonads and adrenal gland. It is used to make synthetic estrogens such as the conjugated or esterified estrogens.
- *Estriol* is an excretory metabolite of estradiol and estrone. It is excreted as a soluble conjugate. Estriol has relatively little estrogenic potency. It is important, however, as an index of normal fetal development (*see* p. 83).

Progesterone
Progesterone is a steroid hormone produced by the corpus luteum after ovulation (*see* Figure 11.3), and by the placenta during pregnancy. Progesterone is essential for pregnancy.

Physiological actions
- Causes a secretory post-ovulatory uterine endothelium
- Increases body temperature

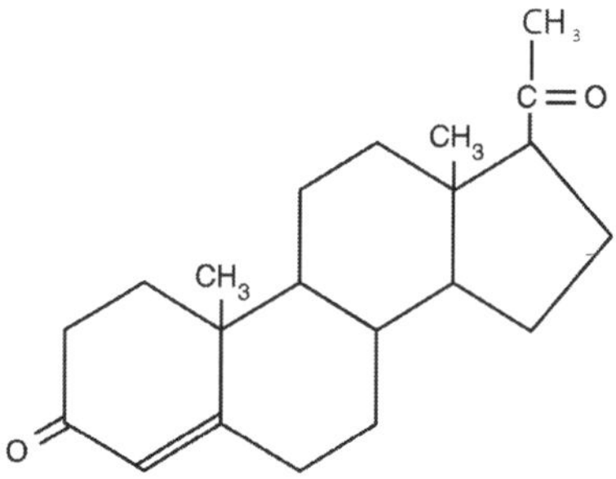

Figure 11.3 The structure of progesterone.

- Stimulates lipoprotein kinase activity
- Enhances fat deposition
- Increases basal insulin levels in blood
- Enhances the sensitivity of cells to insulin
- Enhances the sensitivity of the islets of Langerhans to circulating glucose
- Promotes glycogen storage in the liver
- Promotes ketogenesis
- Essential for pregnancy
- Increases the ventilatory response to CO_2
- Promotes alveolobular development in the breast
- Has depressant and sedating effects on the brain

Examples of synthetic progestogens

- Medroxyprogesterone acetate
- Megestrol acetate
- Norethindrone
- Norgestrel

Therapeutic uses of synthetic progestogens (US: progestins)

- Oral contraception (*see* p. 90)
- HRT
- To arrest precocious puberty

Chapter 11 quiz

Answer T (true) or F (false)

1 Estradiol causes epiphyseal closure at puberty ☐

2 Estradiol is responsible for the female pattern of fat distribution ☐

3 Estradiol inhibits progesterone receptor synthesis ☐

4 In pregnancy, estradiol limits bodily fluid retention ☐

5 Estradiol increases plasma LDL ☐

6 Estradiol enhances fluid retention ☐

7 Estradiol stimulates myometrial oxytocin receptor synthesis ☐

8 Estradiol promotes calcium resorption from bone ☐

9 Estradiol decreases bowel motility ☐

10 SERMs are selective estrogen receptor agonists ☐

11 Aromatase inhibitors block conversion of androgens to estrogens ☐

12 Estrogens are known to worsen breast cancer ☐

13 SERMs and aromatase inhibitors are indicated for estrogen
receptor-positive biopsies ☐

14 Estrogen loss may be implicated in postmenopausal osteoporosis ☐

15 Estrone is a powerful estrogen ☐

A Progesterone:

- Is essential for pregnancy to be maintained ☐
- Is produced by the ovarian follicle before ovulation ☐
- Enhances cellular sensitivity to insulin ☐
- Produces a secretory post-ovulatory uterine endothelium ☐
- Promotes alveolobular development in the breast ☐
- Decreases body temperature ☐

B Can you complete the labelling of this figure?

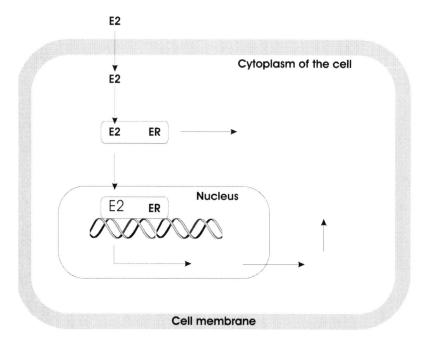

ER, estrogen receptor; E2, estradiol.

12 Endocrinology of pregnancy, parturition and lactation

Learning objectives
Brief glossary of pregnancy and parturition
Major hormones of pregnancy
Parturition
Lactation
Prolactin
The suckling reflex

Learning objectives

- Be able to list the major hormones of pregnancy and know in which tissues they are synthesised and what their major actions are
- Be acquainted with the endocrine events that play an important role in the onset and course of labour
- Be able to give a brief account of the endocrine events implicated in parturition and lactation
- Outline the central events of the suckling reflex

Brief glossary of pregnancy and parturition

- *Blastocyst*: early embryonic stage; a hollow ball of cells with an inner wall thickening which will become the embryo. The rest of the cell lining will become the trophoblast (*see* Figure 12.1)
- *Corpus luteum*: 'yellow body' – disrupted Graafian follicle after rupture at ovulation
- *Fetoplacental unit*: term to describe the reproductive assembly plant, which consists chiefly of the placenta and the fetus
- *Lactation*: milk secretion from the breasts
- *Lactogenesis*: production of milk
- *Parturition*: labour and childbirth
- *Placenta*: organ within the uterus which is the interface between mother and embryo:
  - for supplying nutrients and respiratory gases
  - for eliminating fetal waste products
  - as an endocrine gland, synthesising steroid and protein hormones
- *Post-partum*: after birth has occurred

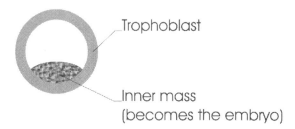

Figure 12.1 The blastocyst.

- *Syncytiotrophoblast*: cells of the trophoblast which lose cellular structure and become a syncytium, i.e. the invasive part of the trophoblast that invades maternal tissue and becomes the villi of the placenta
- *Trimester*: any one of the three-month intervals of pregnancy, i.e. first, second or third trimesters
- *Trophoblast*: tissue forming the walls of the blastocyst

Major hormones of pregnancy

- Progesterone ⎫
- Estriol   ⎭ Steroids
- Human chorionic gonadotrophin (HCG) ⎫
- Human placental lactogen (HPL)   ⎬ Protein hormones
- Relaxin   ⎭

Steroid hormones

Progesterone

Site of biosynthesis in pregnancy
- First trimester: corpus luteum
- Second and third trimesters: placenta

Functions in pregnancy
- Prepares the endometrium for implantation of the blastocyst
- Stimulates endometrial secretions and is necessary for formation of the cervical mucus plug
- Inhibits contractility of the myometrial muscle, which prevents premature abortion
- Important in preparing the mammary glands for lactation

Progesterone levels in the maternal blood stream rise steeply during pregnancy (*see* Figure 12.2(a)).

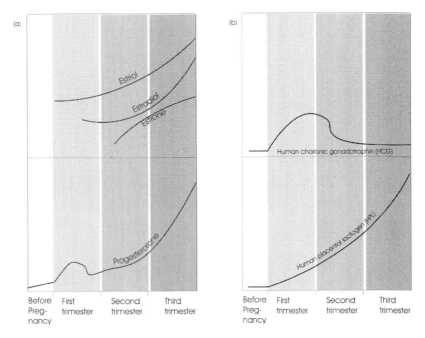

Figure 12.2 (a) Female sex steroids during pregnancy; (b) female protein hormones during pregnancy.

Estrogens
- Estradiol
- Estriol
- Estrone
- All three hormones rise progressively in the maternal circulation during pregnancy (*see* Figure 12.2(b))
- Both mother and fetus are important sources of estrogen precursors (*see* Figure 12.3)

Estriol as a marker of healthy fetal development
- Maternal plasma levels rise during pregnancy (*see* Figure 12.2(a)).
- Maternal plasma levels reflect fetal health because estriol is synthesised by the fetal adrenal gland (*see* Figure 12.3) under the influence of the fetal anterior pituitary ACTH.
- Therefore abnormally low estriol reflects an unhealthy pituitary and therefore interference with normal fetal growth.

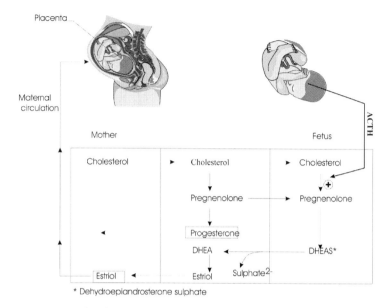

Figure 12.3 Estriol and progesterone biosynthesis in pregnancy. DHEA, dehydroepiandrosterone; DHEAS, dehydroepiandrosterone sulphate.

Protein hormones

Human chorionic gonadotrophin (HCG)

- *Chemical structure*: similar to LH
- *Site of synthesis*: the syncytiotrophoblast; therefore the presence of HCG in maternal urine or blood signals the presence of an embryo (pregnancy test method)
- *Initial detectability*: 8–10 days after fertilisation
- *Functions in pregnancy*:
  - prevents luteolysis, i.e. prevents destruction of the corpus luteum
  - stimulates fetal hormone production, e.g. promotes testosterone production by the male fetus
  - stimulates luteal progesterone production
- *Other uses*:
  - used to mimic the LH surge in infertile women in order to trigger ovulation
  - used to correct luteal phase defects

Human placental lactogen (HPL)

Also known as chorionic somatomammotrophin (HCS)

- *Chemical structure*: similar to GH and prolactin (PRL)

- *Site of synthesis*: the syncytiotrophoblast
- *Initial detectability*: 2–5 weeks after fertilisation; in maternal but not fetal circulation; plasma levels rise with placental growth (*see* Figure 12.2(b))
- *Functions in pregnancy* – controversial, some effects reported:
  - like growth hormone, is diabetogenic
  - involved in mobilisation of free fatty acids
  - involved in maternal glucose metabolism
  - contributes to the phenomenon of insulin resistance noted in pregnancy
  - these metabolic effects contribute to increased availability of amino acids and glucose
  - HPL production is approximately proportional to placental mass
- Seldom detected in plasma of non-pregnant women

Relaxin
- *Chemical structure*: a polypeptide, with 3-dimensional structure similar to that of insulin, but with a different amino acid sequence
- *Sites of biosynthesis*: mainly the corpus luteum, placenta and some by the decidual lining of the uterus
- *Initial detectability*: detectable approximately when HCG levels start to rise and remains detectable throughout pregnancy
- *Actions*: synergistic with progesterone to inhibit uterine contractility; relaxes the connective tissue of the pubic symphysis where the pubic bones fuse, so they can widen to facilitate the birth of the fetus
- *Mechanism of action*: increasing secretion of plasminogen activator and collagenase, enzymes which dissolve collagen

Parturition

What is it?
- Parturition is the onset and course of labour and birth
- *Cause of onset in humans*: unknown; in sheep, parturition is known to be dependent on a rise in fetal cortisol

Endocrine events implicated in onset and course of labour

- Rise in estrogen levels causes increased synthesis in uterus of oxytocin receptors
- Fetus produces relatively large amounts of oxytocin
- Increased release of adrenal cortisol by fetus
- Increased production of prostaglandins PGF_{2a} and PGE_2, possibly stimulated by oxytocin; PGF_{2a} and PGE_2 cause uterine contraction during labour, a steep fall in maternal progesterone and estrogen blood levels, which allows prolactin to stimulate milk production (*see* below)

- Upregulation of the enzyme nitric oxide synthase, part of the system for 'ripening' the cervix to allow passage of the fetus
- At onset of labour, a large influx into the myometrium (uterine smooth muscle) of leucocytes

Lactation

What is it?

Lactation is milk secretion from the breasts, which become enlarged during pregnancy through the action of several hormones, including:

- cortisol
- estrogens
- growth hormone
- HPL
- prolactin (*see* below)
- progesterone.

Prolactin

- *Chemical structure*: a polypeptide of molecular weight about 22 000 Da, containing 198 amino acids
- *Site of biosynthesis*: lactotroph cells of the anterior pituitary gland
- *Control of biosynthesis*: hypothalamic control, mainly inhibitory through the neurotransmitter *dopamine* (also called prolactin-inhibitory factor; PIF); TRH (*see* p. 31) is a powerful releaser of prolactin, and a prolactin-releasing peptide has recently been reported
- *Actions*:
  - post-partum stimulation of milk production
  - suppression of gonadal function, which renders women infertile during suckling; the mechanism appears to be, in part, through suppression of pulsatile GnRH release from the hypothalamus
  - in men, hyperprolactinaemia suppresses spermatogenesis, depresses testosterone production and appears to lower libido
  - prolactin levels are raised in stress
  - prolactin causes hair growth

The suckling reflex

What is it?

The suckling reflex is the reflex letting down of milk, caused by the mechanical stimulation of the nipple (e.g. by the baby's mouth).[1]

---

[1] There is evidence that the sound of the hungry baby's cries will also elicit the suckling reflex.

Mechanism

1   Mechanical stimulation of the nipple sends afferent nerve impulses up the spinal cord to the supraoptic and paraventricular nuclei of the hypo-thalamus.

2   This stimulates oxytocin secretion into the general circulation from the posterior pituitary gland.

3   Oxytocin contracts myoepithelial tissue in the mammary glands and milk is ejected from the nipple.

> *Note:* prolactin is also released into the circulation during the suckling reflex by an as yet poorly understood mechanism.

Chapter 12 quiz

Answer T (true) or F (false)

A Important functions of progesterone in pregnancy are:
- It prepares the endometrium for blastocyst implantation ☐
- It is necessary for formation of the cervical mucus plug ☐
- Stimulation of endometrial secretions ☐
- It enhances the contractility of endometrial muscle ☐
- It has an important role in preparing mammary glands for lactation ☐

B Estriol:
- Maternal plasma levels normally fall as pregnancy progresses ☐
- Is synthesised by the fetal adrenal gland ☐
- Secretion by the fetus is controlled by fetal TRH ☐
- Levels therefore reflect the health of the fetal pituitary ☐

C Human chorionic gonadotrophin (HCG):
- Is structurally related to FSH ☐
- Is an indicator of pregnancy ☐
- Is detected in the second trimester ☐
- Is synthesised by the syncytiotrophoblast ☐
- Prevents destruction of the corpus luteum ☐
- Stimulates luteal progesterone production ☐
- Stimulates testosterone production by the fetus ☐

D Human placental lactogen (HPL):
- Is structurally similar to growth hormone and prolactin ☐
- Is synthesised by the corpus luteum ☐
- Is initially detected 2–5 weeks after fertilisation in fetal blood ☐
- Reported effects include:
  - diabetogenic ☐
  - contributes to insulin resistance of pregnancy ☐
  - increased availability of amino acids and glucose ☐

E Relaxin:
- Is structurally similar to insulin ☐
- Is synthesised mainly in the decidual lining of the uterus ☐
- Is initially detected when HCG levels start to rise ☐
- Synergises with progesterone to inhibit uterine motility ☐
- Relaxes connective tissue of the pubic symphysis at birth ☐

F Parturition:
- Is the onset and course of labour and birth ☐

- In humans is initiated by a rise in fetal cortisol
- Is associated with increased oxytocin production by the fetus
- Is facilitated by increased uterine contractility
- Is accompanied by a sharp fall in plasma progesterone
- Is accompanied by a sharp rise in nitric oxide synthase activity

G Prolactin:
- Is synthesised by lactotroph cells in the posterior pituitary
- Release is stimulated by dopamine
- Stimulates milk production in the breast
- Suppresses fertility during suckling
- Levels are raised in stress
- Suppresses testosterone synthesis and spermatogenesis

13 Contraception

Learning objectives

- Be able to list the different approved contraceptive methods available and important points when choosing one
- Know what types of combined oral contraceptive pills (COCPs) are available and be able to give an example of each
- Be aware of the mechanism of action of the COCP
- Be able to list advantages, adverse effects, risks and contraindications of COCP usage
- Know examples of the progestogen-only pill (POP), and be able to list advantages and disadvantages of the POP
- Know the given disadvantages, risks and limitations of emergency contraception
- Be able to give a brief account of the available IUDs, their advantages, disadvantages, adverse effects, precautions and contraindications
- Be aware of the nature of other, non-chemical contraceptive methods

Choosing a contraceptive method: some important points to consider

- Seeking medical advice
- Effectiveness of the method
- Known risks and adverse effects of the method
- Whether a future pregnancy is being planned

- Existing medically treated conditions
- Personal preferences and partner relationship status

Contraceptive methods dealt with in this chapter

- Combined oral contraceptive pill (COCP)
- Progestogen[1]-only pill (POP)
- Contraceptive implants
- Contraceptive injections
- Transdermal patches
- Barrier methods
- Intrauterine devices (IUDs)
- Hormone-releasing intra-uterine devices
- Emergency contraceptives
- Vasectomy
- Fertility awareness

The combined oral contraceptive pill (COCP)

- *Active constituents*: an estrogen and a progestogen

Types of COCP

- *Monophasic*:
    - *fixed low estrogen dose* + progestogen in each tablet, e.g. ethinylestradiol 20 µg; norethisterone acetate 1mg; 21 tablets (Loestrin20® Galen Pharmaceuticals)
    - *fixed standard estrogen dose* + progestogen in each tablet, e.g. ethinyl-estradiol 30 µg; levonorgestrel 150 µg; 21 tablets (Microgynon 30® Schering Health)
- *Diphasic and triphasic*: varying doses of estrogen and progestogen to mimic hormone changes during the menstrual cycle

Mechanism of action

- Estrogen inhibits FSH release from the anterior pituitary, which prevents follicle development, and progestogen inhibits preovulatory LH surge.
- Progestogen also changes cervical mucus consistency, which prevents spermatozoa from penetrating an ovum that may have been released.

Efficacy

If properly used, efficacy is estimated at 99.9%.

[1] USA: progestin

Deciding on choice of COCP

Decisions are made largely on the dose of estrogen:

- low strength, e.g. ethinylestradiol 20 µg
- standard strength, e.g. ethinylestradiol 30–40 µg (increased risk of venous thromboembolism).

Advantages of the COCP

- The most effective method
- May reduce risks of:
  - endometrial, colonic and ovarian epithelial cancer with long-term usage
  - rheumatoid arthritis and osteoporosis
  - benign ovarian tumours, symptoms of dysmenorrhoea and acne
- Little delay in return to fertility after stopping the COCP
- COCPs may be administered as transdermal patches, which reduces greatly the risks of missing a dose (see the *British National Formulary* (*BNF*) for example)

Adverse effects

Adverse effects usually occur within the first 1–3 months of treatment, after which they may subside:

- breakthrough bleeding
- nausea, vomiting, diarrhoea
- weight gain (salt and water retention)
- headaches (possibly from hypertension).

Drug interactions

The efficacy of both estrogen and progestogen may be reduced through accelerated metabolism due to induction of liver microsomal enzymes by (e.g.):[2]

- antivirals
- antitubercular drugs rifabutin and rifampicin (powerful interaction)
- anti-epileptic drugs e.g. phenobarbital, carbamazepine.

Risks associated with COCP use[3]

COCP use is associated with an increased risk of:

- haemorrhagic and ischaemic stroke

---

[2] This list is not comprehensive.
[3] Familial history of cardiovascular disease and malignancy is an important risk factor with COCPs.

- myocardial infarction and stroke in older women and heavy smokers
- ischaemic stroke in asthma patients, migraine sufferers, hypertension; increased if all coupled with smoking
- breast cancer (less with low dose COCPs)
- venous thromboembolism (VTE) in:
    - older women
    - smokers
    - obesity
    - post-surgery
    - thrombophilia
    - malignancy
    - use of COCPs containing desogestrel or gestodene
    - family history of VTE
    - varicose veins
    - immobilisation
- cervical cancer with more than 5 years' use
- liver cancer with long-term use
- breast cancer with higher-dose estrogen COCPs
- diabetes mellitus in arterial disease.

COCPs do not protect against sexually transmitted diseases.

Contraindications for COCPs[4]

- Pregnancy
- Personal history of cardiovascular disorders, e.g. VTE, stroke, hypertension, arterial or venous thrombosis
- Migraine
- Systemic lupus erythematosus (SLE)
- Liver disease
- Malignancy
- Undiagnosed vaginal bleeding
- During breast-feeding
- Gonadotrophin-secreting tumour

Progesterone

- *Active constituent*: synthetic progestogen
- *Indications for use*: women for whom estrogens are contraindicated, e.g. predisposition to or history of venous thrombosis, smokers, diabetics and migraine sufferers, and for patients with hypertension or valvular disease

---

[4] This list is not comprehensive; see *BNF*.

The progestogen-only pill

Preparations and dosage

- Oral progestogens used include:
  - *desogestrel* 28 × 75 mg (Cerazette® Organon)
  - *etynodiol diacetate* 28 × 500 µg (Femulen® Pharmacia)
  - *levonorgestrel* 35 × 30 µg (Microval® Wyeth)
  - *norethisterone* 28 × 350 µg (Micronor® Jannsen-Cilag)
- *Administration*: usually one tablet daily, starting on day 1 of the menstrual cycle

---

Note: oral POPs should be taken at the same time each day, as a delay of even 3 hours could compromise contraceptive cover.

Contraindications with POPs

- History of breast cancer, but may be used if there is no recurrence after 5 years
- Pregnancy
- Undiagnosed vaginal bleeding
- Liver disorders, e.g. liver adenoma
- Porphyria
- Gonadotrophin-secreting tumours

Risks associated with POP use

- Ectopic pregnancy if POP taken at time of fertilisation
- Benign ovarian cysts

Parenteral progestogens

Parenteral[5] progestogens used include:

- *medroxyprogesterone acetate* (Depo-Provera® Pharmacia) as a pre-filled 1 ml syringe containing 150 mg of medroxyprogesterone acetate for deep IM injection
  - *timing of administration*: 5 days after parturition (birth) or delayed for 6 weeks if breast-feeding. Added contraceptive cover, e.g. barrier method, should be used for 14 days after injection. Length of cover about 12 weeks
- *norethisterone enantate* (Noristerat® Schering Health) as an oily injection containing 200 mg in 1 ml, for slow injection into the gluteal muscle

---

[5] Professional advice and professional product administration are essential, as well as consultation of the product's literature before use.

- *timing of administration*: within 5 days of the cycle or immediately after parturition. Mothers who take this treatment should not breast-feed babies with persistent or severe jaundice that requires medical treatment. The length of cover is 8 weeks
- *etonogestrel* (Implanon® Organon) as an implant containing 68 mg in a flexible rod for subdermal insertion during the first 5 days of the menstrual cycle:
  - *timing of administration*: it may be implanted between days 21 and 28 after abortion or birth; if it is implanted after 28 days, additional precautions to prevent fertilisation are recommended.

Advantages of parenteral progestogen contraception

- Avoids problem of missed doses
- May alleviate premenstrual syndrome, dysmenorrhoea and pelvic pain
- May protect against pelvic infection through the barrier effect of a progestogen-induced cervical mucus plug
- Use not contraindicated during breast-feeding

Disadvantages of parenteral progestogen contraception

- Progestogen injection is irreversible; adverse effects may persist until dose is eliminated
- Return of fertility after injection wears off is variable, and fertility may be delayed for several months
- Menses may become light or cease altogether until the effects of the drug wear off

Adverse effects of progesterone

- Nausea, vomiting
- Breast discomfort, menstrual irregularities and 'spotting' between periods
- Central effects, e.g. headache, depression, mild sedation (derivatives of progesterone have been developed as general anaesthetics), dizziness, loss of libido
- Appetite and weight changes
- Skin disorders

Emergency contraception

This is the use (in the UK) of levonorgestrel within 32 hours of having unprotected sexual intercourse. The sooner the dose is taken the better the chances of blocking fertilisation.

Disadvantages

- Requirement for a prescription

- Lower efficiency than IUDs
- Possibility of vomiting after taking the dose
- Possible interference with timing of the next menstruation
- A possibility of an ectopic pregnancy (symptoms include lower abdominal pain)
- Need for barrier contraception until the next menses
- Drug interactions, e.g. enzyme-inducing drugs will reduce the efficacy of levonorgestrel

Intrauterine devices (IUDs)

- Intra-uterine progestogen-only devices
- Intra-uterine copper-based devices

Mechanism note: progestogen-based IUDs thicken cervical mucus to hinder penetration of spermatozoa and create an endometrium hostile to implantation of a fertilised ovum. Copper-based IUDs induce a sterile anti-inflammatory reaction in the uterus, which changes uterine and fallopian tube fluid composition, which in turn destroys the viability of both the ovum and the spermatozoa. The progestogen-based IUD probably acts through a combination of both hormonal- and inflammation-based reactions.

Intra-uterine progestogen-only devices

- *Levonorgestrel* (Mirena® Schering Health) is a T-shaped plastic device containing levonorgestrel released directly into the uterine cavity at a rate which is aimed to release 24 µg every 24 hours. In the UK it is licensed for use as a contraceptive for prevention of endometrial hyperplasia during estrogen HRT and for treatment of primary menorrhagia.
- *Timing of administration*: insert into the uterine cavity
  - within 7 days of onset of menses, although it can be inserted at any time if it is a replacement
  - immediately after first-trimester termination by curettage[6]
  - 6 weeks after childbirth.
- Contraception is claimed to be effective for 5 years after insertion.

Advantages

- Long period of effectiveness
- Reduced risk of drug interactions

---

[6] Curettage: physical removal of debris, usually by suction, after cleansing a diseased surface with a curet (curved spoon); used in first-trimester abortion.

- Rapid restoration of fertility after removal
- Hormonal effects are local
- Useful for women who have heavy menses; significant reduction in bleeding in women with primary menorrhagia
- Reduced frequency of pelvic inflammatory disease
- Device may have additional contraceptive action
- Lower incidence of side-effects than with other intra-uterine devices (*see* below)

Adverse effects, precautions and contraindications[7]

These are generally as for other fitted IUDs (*see* below).

- Occasional development of functional ovarian cysts
- Abdominal pain, oedema, migraine, hirsutism, mood changes may occur
- Risk of cervical/uterine perforation if not fitted properly by qualified personnel
- Check for sexually transmitted diseases before use

Contraindications

Contraindications for any intra-uterine device include pregnancy, severe anaemia, untreated sexually transmitted diseases, small or distorted uterus, undiagnosed or unexplained uterine bleeding and malignancy of the genitourinary tract.

Copper-based intra-uterine devices

- *Flexi-T*® *300* (*FP*): copper wire wound onto the vertical stem of a T-shaped frame and impregnated with barium sulphate to give the device radio-opacity
- *GyneFix*® (*FP*): copper sleeves on polypropylene thread (no frame)
- *Multiload*® *Cu375*(*Organon*): copper wire wound onto the vertical stem of a device with two flexible U-shaped side-arms
- *NovaT*® *380* (*Schering Health*): similar design to *Flexi-T*®
- *T-Safe*® *Cu280A* (*FP*): similar design to *Flexi-T*® *300* but with copper collars on the distal end of each arm

Other contraceptive devices

- Contraceptive caps
- Contraceptive diaphragms
- Male and female condoms

[7] This is not a comprehensive list; those who wish to use an IUD should discuss their particular medical status with a clinician first.

Contraceptive diaphragms and caps

- Need to be fitted by a professional, but thereafter can be inserted personally
- Need practice to use
- Freely available from clinics
- If used with a spermicide, about 98% effective

Male and female condoms

- Male condom calculated as 98% effective
- Female condom ('femidom') calculated as 95% effective
- Freely available from clinics and vending machines
- May give protection from sexually transmittable infections (STIs), but should not be regarded as a completely reliable safeguard from STIs, as condoms may tear, leak or be displaced

Natural methods of contraception

These involve constant monitoring of personal fertility status, by measuring body temperature, which rises measurably after ovulation, and by observing cervical secretions, since the nature of secretions changes during the menstrual cycle. Advantages are avoidance of artificial contraception with its attendant risks, and regular personal monitoring of reproductive function. Disadvantages include the need for professional instruction and a delay while the process is learned.

Male/female sterilisation

- *Male sterilisation* involves vasectomy to block passage of spermatozoa. Advantages include reversibility of the operation and freedom from condom use (but this increases the risk of STIs).
- *Female sterilisation* involves prevention of the ovum from passing through the fallopian tubes. A disadvantage is that a general anaesthetic is required both to initiate and reverse the contraception.

Chapter 13 quiz

Answer T (true) or F (false)

1 Monophasic oral contraceptives have a variable estrogen dose ☐
2 Monophasic oral contraceptives have fixed doses of estrogen + progestogen ☐
3 Estrogen's contraceptive action is through blocking LH release ☐
4 Progestogens inhibit preovulatory LH release ☐
5 Progestogen changes cervical mucus consistency ☐
6 The COCP efficacy is estimated to be 95% ☐
7 Higher doses of estrogen are associated with an increased risk of venous thromboembolism ☐
8 COCPs may reduce the risks of colonic, endometrial and epithelial cancers ☐
9 Oral contraceptive efficacy may be reduced by drugs which induce liver microsomal enzymes, e.g. rifampicin ☐
10 Low-dose COCPs do not reduce the risk of breast cancer ☐
11 Combined COCPs used for more than 5 years may increase cervical cancer risk ☐
12 There is no risk of liver cancer with long-term use ☐
13 There is increased risk of breast cancer with COCPs ☐

A Adverse effects of combined COCPs (especially within the first 3 months) include:
- Weight gain ☐
- Breakthrough bleeding ☐
- Diarrhoea, nausea and vomiting ☐
- Headache ☐
- Dysmenorrhoea ☐

B Risks associated with the COCP include:
- Myocardial infarction and stroke in older women and smokers ☐
- Ischaemic stroke and haemorrhage ☐
- Risks of ischaemic stroke in smokers ☐
- Venous thromboembolism in women:
  - who smoke ☐
  - who are older ☐
  - after surgery ☐
  - who are obese ☐
  - with malignancy ☐

C The progestogen-only pill:
- Cannot be prescribed for women in whom the COCP is contraindicated ☐
- Should be taken at the same time each day to maximise contraceptive cover ☐
- May increase ectopic pregnancy risk if taken at time of fertilisation ☐

- May cause appetite and weight changes ☐
- May have central effects, e.g. mild sedation, dizziness ☐
- Is associated with increased risk of benign ovarian cysts ☐
- Is contraindicated in:
  - pregnancy ☐
  - porphyria ☐
  - undiagnosed vaginal bleeding ☐
  - gonadotrophin-secreting tumours ☐
  - liver disorders, e.g. liver adenoma ☐
  - if there is no recurrence of breast cancer after 5 years ☐

D   Advantages of parenteral progestogen contraception are:
- It avoids the problem of missing a dose ☐
- It may alleviate problems, e.g. PMS, dysmenorrhoea ☐
- It reduces pelvic infection risks ☐
- There is a rapid return to fertility after the injection wears off ☐

E   Disadvantages of emergency contraception include:
- Danger of an ectopic pregnancy ☐
- A prescription is needed ☐
- It is less effective than an IUD ☐
- It can cause nausea and vomiting (with loss of drug) ☐
- It may change the timing of the next menses ☐
- Need for barrier contraception until the following menses ☐
- Reduced efficacy if taken with enzyme-inducing drugs ☐

F   Advantages of progestogen-only IUDs are:
- They can be used in pregnancy ☐
- A long period of contraceptive cover ☐
- Rapid restoration of fertility after removal ☐
- Virtually all hormonal effects are local ☐
- They reduce the risk of pelvic inflammatory disease ☐
- They are an option for women with heavy menses ☐

14   Can you list the contraindications for COCPs?

14 The menopause and hormone replacement therapy

Learning objectives
Important endocrine changes at menopause
Timing and symptoms of menopause
Health risks associated with menopause
Treatment
Hormone replacement therapy
Osteoporosis

Learning objectives

- Know what menopause is and its symptoms and effects
- Have knowledge of the various HRT options, their adverse effects, contraindications and risks
- Know the names of treatments available for osteoporosis associated with menopause

---

Definition

Menopause is cessation of menstruation.

Important endocrine changes at menopause

- Failure of ovaries to respond to normal anterior pituitary hormones, e.g. LH and FSH
- Reduction and eventual cessation of ovarian steroid hormone production
- Cessation of ovulation and of the menstrual cycle
- Loss of fertility

Timing and symptoms of menopause

The nature, timing and severity of menopausal symptoms vary with the individual; some women have virtually no symptoms while others may need both medicinal and psychosocial support. Menopause usually occurs after 50 years, but can (albeit relatively rarely) occur 10 years earlier. Onset may be gradual with irregularity of menstrual occurrence, and menopause is generally accepted as cessation of menses for 12 months. Symptoms include:

- emotional changes and mood swings
- cardiovascular symptoms, e.g. tachycardia and arrhythmias and symptoms of generalised vasodilation, including headaches and 'hot flushes'
- androgenic symptoms, e.g. facial and body hair growth
- pain in joints
- insomnia and fatigue
- dry itchy skin and genital discomfort due to decreased mucosal secretions
- vaginal atrophy and increased risk of vaginal infection
- increased risk of urinary infections and urinary incontinence
- loss of skin firmness and plasticity
- osteoporosis (bone loss with increased fracture risk).

Health risks associated with menopause

- Weakness of the pelvic floor due to gradual weakening of the pelvic joints and muscles, increasing the risk of uterine prolapse[1]
- Raised cholesterol LDL levels, thus increasing chances of cardiovascular disease, e.g. hypertension, atherosclerosis and stroke
- Weight gain
- Osteoporosis and bone density loss, thus increasing fracture risk
- Emotional problems e.g. depression

Treatment

Treatment options include:

- hormone replacement therapy (HRT)
- diet and exercise
- prevention and treatment of osteoporosis
- counselling.

Hormone replacement therapy

Aim of treatment

To prevent or reduce the incidence and severity of menopausal symptoms associated with the loss of natural estrogens and progesterone.

Main treatments used

- *Low-dose estrogen*: e.g. natural estradiol, synthetic ethinylestradiol
- *Low dose estrogen + a synthetic progestogen*: e.g. estradiol valerate + norethisterone
- *Combined conjugated estrogens*[2] alone or + a progestogen

[1] Uterine prolapse: the uterus drops into the vaginal region.
[2] Conjugated here means a mixture of naturally occurring estrogen sulphates (mainly) extracted from urine of pregnant mares.

- *Progestogen* alone
- *Tibolone*, a steroid combining estrogenic, progestogenic and androgenic actions
- *Raloxifene*, an estrogen receptor modulator, for prevention and treatment of postmenopausal osteoporosis (*see* also below); raloxifene does not block other postmenopausal cardiovascular symptoms such as hot flushes

Choice of HRT treatment[3]

Choice of HRT depends on:

- the patient's reproductive organ status, i.e. the presence or absence of a uterus; low-dose estrogen alone may be considered suitable in a patient without a uterus
- patient tolerance to the drug and adverse effects
- the preferred route of administration: patients may not tolerate oral administration, when a patch may be more suitable, and more convenient for the patient.

Currently, tibolone is the most widely prescribed HRT for women who have not undergone hysterectomy.

Routes of administration of HRT

- *Oral*, e.g. low-dose synthetic estrogens or conjugated estrogens, either alone or with progestogens
- *Patches* containing natural estradiol alone or together with a synthetic progestogen
- *Vaginal rings* containing estradiol
- *Gels* containing estradiol for topical application
- *Nasal sprays* containing estradiol

Adverse effects of HRT[4]

- *Estrogenic effects*: e.g. weight gain, headaches, cramps in legs, fluid retention, nausea, breast tenderness
- *Progestogenic effects*: e.g. constipation and bloating sensations, symptoms of premenstrual tension
- *Other effects*: e.g. occasionally cholelithiasis (formation of stones in the gall bladder), hypertension, occasionally impaired glucose tolerance, contact lens discomfort, epistaxis (nosebleeds)

Contraindications to HRT

- Estrogen-dependent breast cancer

---

[3] Choice should always be made with the help of professional medical advice.

[4] This list is not exhaustive.

- Dubin–Johnson and Rotor's syndromes[5]
- Patient history of venous thrombosis
- Recent or current arterial thromboembolic disorders, e.g. angina or myocardial infarction
- Active thrombophlebitis
- Untreated endometrial hyperplasia
- Undiagnosed vaginal bleeding
- Pregnancy and breast-feeding

HRT (or oral contraceptives) should also be avoided in patients with hepatic (liver) disease.

Main risks associated with HRT

- Venous thromboembolism and stroke
- Endometrial cancer (although risk is lessened with progestogen use)
- Increased risk of breast cancer within 1–2 years after starting HRT; risk may lessen within 5 years of stopping HRT use
- Increased risk of liver damage and gallstones if used for more than 5 years
- Estrogen-alone HRT is associated generally with more risk than low-dose estrogen combined with a progestogen

Osteoporosis

What is osteoporosis?

Osteoporosis is the loss of bone tissue, resulting in brittle, excessively porous bones that are liable to fractures with infection. Postmenopausal osteoporosis is, to a large extent, due to the loss of estrogens, and HRT is used to counteract bone loss.

Drugs used to treat postmenopausal osteopososis

- Raloxifene
- Hormonal HRT
- Bisphosphonates:
  - alendronic acid
  - disodium etidronate
  - risedronate
- Calcitonin (*see* also p. 191) for patients who cannot tolerate bisphosphonates

---

[5] Dubin–Johnson syndrome: very rare autosomal recessive inherited disorder resulting in mild lifelong jaundice. Rotor's syndrome: a rare idiopathic form of hyperbilirubinaemia.

Chapter 14 quiz
Answer T (true) or F (false)

A   Menopause:
- Is interruption of menstruation
- Is cessation of menstruation
- Always has an onset after 50 years of age
- Is accompanied by reduction and eventual failure of sex hormone production
- May be caused in part by failure of the ovaries to respond to LH and FSH

B   Symptoms of menopause may include:
- Cardiovascular symptoms, e.g. 'hot flushes' and arrhythmias
- Calcification of bone
- Vaginal dryness and atrophy
- Hardening of skin due to cornification
- Mood swings
- Joint pain, fatigue and insomnia
- Urinary incontinence and increased urinary infection risk
- Weight loss
- Increased LDL with raised atherosclerosis risk

C   Hormone replacement therapy (HRT) includes:
- Treatment for hypercalcaemia
- Sex hormone replacement
- Counselling
- Bed rest

D   The main HRT treatments are:
- Low-dose estrogen
- Low-dose estrogen + a progestogen
- Glucocorticoids
- Combined conjugated estrogens
- Progestogen alone
- Tibolone

E   The main routes of HRT administration are:
- Nasal sprays containing estradiol
- Topical gels containing estradiol
- Vaginal rings containing estradiol
- Oral low-dose anti-estrogens alone or with a progestogen
- Skin patches containing estradiol, the natural estrogen alone, or with a synthetic progestogen

F   Who should not take HRT?
- Patients who are pregnant or breast-feeding ☐
- Those with undiagnosed vaginal bleeding ☐
- Patients with liver disease ☐
- Patients with acne ☐
- Patients with active thrombophlebitis ☐
- Patients with untreated endometrial hyperplasia ☐
- Patients with a history of venous thrombosis ☐
- Patients with any current or recent thromboembolic arterial disorders, e.g. angina or myocardial infarction ☐
- Patients with Dubin–Johnson or Rotor's syndromes ☐

G   The main risks associated with HRT are:
- Increased risk of endometrial cancer with the combined estrogen–progestogen pill ☐
- Venous thromboembolism and stroke ☐
- Increased breast cancer risk within 1–2 years after starting HRT ☐
- Increased risk of gallstones and liver damage if used for more than 5 years ☐

15 Female reproductive pathophysiology: a glossary

Learning objective
Glossary

Learning objective

- Read through the glossary until able to remember and explain briefly the conditions described

Glossary

Amenorrhoea

Absence of menses (menstruation)

- *Primary amenorrhoea*: no menses onset by age 16; causes include:
  - gonadal dysgenesis with Turner's syndrome[1]
  - true or pseudohermaphroditism
  - gonadal chemotherapy or radiotherapy (*see* also below)
  - polycystic ovary syndrome
- *Secondary amenorrhoea*: no menses for 6 months or more after previously regular menses
- *Hypothalamic amenorrhoea*: caused by disturbances to hypothalamic–pituitary axis, e.g. through excess weight loss (exercise or anorexia nervosa) or stress-related
- *Oligomenorrhoea*: infrequent menses

Dysmenorrhoea

Painful menstruation

- *Spasmodic or primary*: lower abdominal cramp just before and during menstruation, often with associated nausea, syncope, headaches, i.e. symptoms of vasodilation; usually presents with first menses
- *Congestive* (secondary): more common in older women; lower abdominal cramps starting a week or two before menses; may be caused by IUDs, endometriosis, fibroids or by other pelvic inflammatory problems

[1] Turner's syndrome: genetic defect where only one X chromosome is present.

Endometriosis

Ectopic development of endometrial-like tissue in the pelvis; some sites affected may include the ovaries, fallopian tubes, cervix and vagina; surgery may be required

Endometritis

Endometrial inflammation due to infection

Ovarian cancer

Malignant tumour of the ovary, most commonly in postmenopausal women; most often a carcinoma[2]; early detection is difficult as this stage is usually symptom-free; by the time of detection the prognosis is generally poor because of metastasis

Ovarian cysts

Fluid-filled sacs in the ovary, usually benign but capable of swelling and causing abdominal pain; surgery may be indicated; malignancy may develop, and may not be detected until too late for successful treatment

Polycystic ovary syndrome (PCOS)

Failure of Graafian follicle development in the ovary due to LH deficiency; this leads to multiple ovarian cysts; associated with adrenal hyperplasia (*see* p. 51); consequences include infertility and symptoms of androgen excess such as acne and hirsutism; others include obesity and reduced plasma HDL due to hyperinsulinaemia

Postpartum depression

Also known as puerperal depression, postnatal depression, postpartum 'blues': period of sadness and sometimes weeping episodes soon after parturition that usually resolves spontaneously, but which in about 0.01% of cases may require hospitalisation and treatment for depression

Premature ovarian failure

Failure of the ovaries to function properly, i.e. produce ova; usually genetic in origin:

- *genetically determined gonadal dysgenesis*, i.e. failure of ovaries to develop properly; often due to X chromosome abnormalities
- *enzyme defects in steroidogenic pathways*, e.g. 17-hydroxylase deficiency (*see* p. 51)

---

[2] Carcinoma: cancer arising in epithelial tissue.

- *galactosaemia*: abnormally high galactose in children causes failure to thrive and appears to be toxic to developing ovaries
- *autoimmune reactions*: hypothyroidism is often associated with ovarian failure; in some women, ovarian failure is associated with raised circulating antibodies to ovarian-sourced antigens
- *iatrogenic*[3] *ovarian failure*: ovarian failure may result from radio- or chemotherapy for childhood malignancies
- *viral oophoritis*: some cases of ovarian failure may be a consequence of a childhood viral infection, e.g. mumps
- *idiopathic*[4] *ovarian failure*: many cases of ovarian failure occur without an identifiable cause; environmental toxins or occult[5] viral oophoritis may be implicated

Premenstrual tension (premenstrual stress)

Emotional disturbances appearing up to 10 days before the start of menses; symptoms may include uncharacteristic irritability, nervousness, headache, depression and explosive temper; symptoms usually disappear soon after menses starts; the cause is unknown but may involve salt and water retention

Uterine fibroids

Benign tumours of muscular and fibrous tissues in the uterine muscle wall; fibroids may cause pain and discomfort, and excessive menstrual bleeding; fibroids reduce the chances of a successful pregnancy

---

[3] Iatrogenic describes a medical condition caused by a medical treatment or surgical intervention.

[4] Unknown aetiology.

[5] Occult: levels below detection methods; oophoritis is inflammation on or in the ovary.

16 Male reproductive endocrinology

Learning objectives
Male reproductive organs
Testosterone and its major androgenic metabolite
dihydrotestosterone (5α-DHT)
Male reproductive pathophysiology (an abridged
summary)
Treatments

Learning objectives

- Be able to list and describe the main functions of the male reproductive organs
- Be able to reproduce a basic sketch showing their arrangement
- Know the chemical nature and main actions of testosterone and its metabolite dihydrotestosterone (5α-DHT)
- Be able to list the reasons for male infertility and the various treatments
- Know the meanings of the terms gynaecomastia, sperm autoimmunity, impotence and priapism
- Be able to give a brief account of benign prostatic hyperplasia (BPH) and prostate cancer and their respective treatments

Male reproductive organs (see Figure 16.1)

The penis

- Male sexual organ of reproduction, containing the terminal (distal) portion of the urethra, through which semen and urine are ejected from the body
- Becomes erect during sexual excitement due to engorgement with blood, enabling penetration of the vagina
- Physical stimulation in this condition causes a paroxysm of emotion (orgasm) and the ejaculation of semen

The testes

- Male sexual organs of reproduction, consisting mainly of
  - the seminiferous tubules, which respond to the anterior pituitary hormone FSH by producing spermatozoa

- Leydig cells, which respond to the anterior pituitary hormone LH to produce male sex hormones (androgens), principally testosterone
- Need to be external to the body at a lower temperature for spermatozoa production and storage

The epididymis

- Convoluted tube connecting the testes to the vas deferens
- Spermatozoa are stored in the lower part of the epididymis until ejaculation occurs

Vas deferens

- Plural *vasa deferentia*; they occur as a pair of ducts
- The vasa deferentia conduct the spermatozoa from the epididymis to the urethra during ejaculation
- Vasectomy is surgical interruption of flow for male contraceptive purposes and is reversible

Prostate gland

- Male accessory sex gland situated just below the bladder
- Opens into the urethra: during ejaculation it discharges the prostatic fluid, which contributes to the composition of the semen, into the urethra

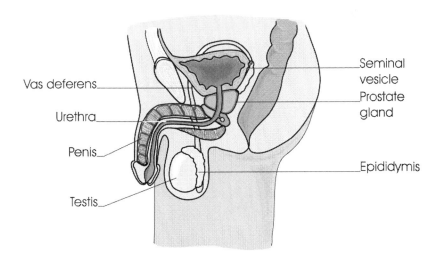

Figure 16.1 The male genital system.

Cowper's glands

- Pair of small glands that open into the urethra at the base of the penis
- They produce part of the seminal fluid

Seminal vesicles

- Pair of accessory male sex glands that produce most of the liquid of the semen; they open into the vas deferens before it joins up with the urethra

Testosterone and its major androgenic metabolite dihydrotestosterone (5α-DHT)

The major androgenic steroid hormones (androgens) cause development and maintenance of male sex organ function, notably:

- spermatogenesis
- maintenance of the accessory sex organs
- male secondary characteristics, which are:
  - voice deepening
  - beard growth
  - skeletal muscle development
  - hair loss.

Other actions of androgens

- Closure of the epiphyses
- Anabolic actions
- Negative feedback effect on gonadotrophin release from the anterior pituitary gland
- Poorly understood actions in the brain affecting brain development both *in utero* and postnatally
- Poorly understood actions in the brain affecting sexual and aggressive behaviour

Male reproductive pathophysiology (an abridged summary)

- *Male infertility* due to:
  - developmental abnormalities
  - primary hypogonadism due to failure of normal testicular development
  - androgen insensitivity due to mutations of the androgen receptor resulting in poor ability (partial insensitivity) or complete failure to bind testosterone (complete insensitivity)

- – gonadotrophin (LH and FSH) deficiencies: secondary hypogonadism, due to e.g. hypothalamic–pituitary disease or anabolic steroid abuse
  - – genital tract obstruction caused by e.g. STIs, vasectomy, bronchiectasis
- *Gynaecomastia*: breast development due to abnormally high estrogen activity
- *Autoimmunity*: sperm autoimmunity when the sperm fail to penetrate the cervical mucus
- *Impotence*: failure of erection due to inadequate blood flow
- *Priapism*: persistent painful penile erection
- *Prostatic pathophysiology*:
  - – benign prostatic hyperplasia
  - – prostate cancer

Treatments

- *Primary hypogonadism*: androgen replacement therapy
- *Androgen insensitivity*: remove testes to prevent possible future carcinogenesis; elective surgery to lengthen vagina + estrogen replacement + community health advice and support
- *Secondary hypogonadism*: gonadotrophin replacement therapy; cease steroid abuse if relevant
- *Autoimmunity*: intracytoplasmic sperm injection, which involves direct injection of a male donor sperm into a donor female egg under the microscope
- *Impotence*: treatment with a vasodilator e.g. sildenafil (*Viagra*®; Pfizer)
- *Priapism*: drain blood from the corpora cavernosa of the penis + apply a vasoconstrictor
- *Benign prostatic hyperplasia*: surgery; alpha-blockers e.g. doxazocin; androgen receptor blockers e.g. finasteride (*Proscar*®; (MSD))
- *Prostate cancer*: ablative surgery, chemotherapy; radiotherapy, cryotherapy; surgical castration; chemical castration with implants of GnRH analogues

---

Mechanism note: pulsatile release (normal ~ hourly) of GnRH from the hypothalamus to the anterior pituitary gland is essential to maintain fertility, but continuous application of GnRH or synthetic analogues shuts down pituitary production of LH and FSH, thus causing a chemical and therefore reversible castration.

Chapter 16 quiz

Answer T (true) or F (false)

1 Androgens exert a positive feedback effect on gonadotrophin release from the anterior pituitary gland ☐

2 5α-dihydrotestosterone is a potent androgenic metabolite of testosterone ☐

3 The Leydig cells of the testis produce the spermatozoa ☐

4 Testosterone is necessary for maintenance of the accessory sex organs ☐

5 The vas deferens conducts spermatozoa from the epididymis to the urethra ☐

6 The Cowper's glands produce part of the seminal fluid ☐

7 Androgens also are anabolic ☐

8 Benign prostatic hyperplasia is treated with radiotherapy ☐

9 Can you label this?

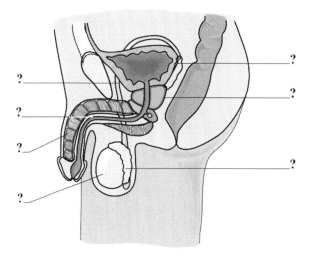

A The penis:
- Ejects semen through the proximal portion of the urethra ☐
- Becomes erect during sexual excitement through engorgement with blood ☐
- Needs to be removed in prostate cancer ☐

B The testes:
- Need to be external to the body at a lower temperature to ensure the viability of the spermatozoa ☐
- Contain Leydig cells which respond to pituitary FSH to synthesise testosterone ☐
- Contain seminiferous tubules which produce the spermatozoa under the influence of FSH ☐

C   Androgens, e.g. testosterone:
- Are necessary for spermatogenesis
- Cause the development of the male sex organs
- Are necessary for maintenance of the sex organs
- Promote scalp hair growth
- Cause voice deepening
- Promote muscle wasting

17 Oxytocin and vasopressin

Learning objectives
Chemical nature and biosynthesis of oxytocin
Physiological actions of oxytocin
Control of oxytocin biosynthesis and release and
*   oxytocin receptor production*
Mechanism of action of oxytocin
Chemical nature, biosynthesis and secretion of
*   vasopressin*
Actions of vasopressin
Pathophysiology of vasopressin

Learning objectives

- Know that oxytocin and vasopressin are both nonapeptides and their sites and manner of production and release
- Be able to list important physiological actions of oxytocin and vasopressin and the factors that promote their release
- Be ready to describe the factors that control oxytocin and vasopressin release and mechanisms of action
- Know the consequences of failed vasopressin release and the treatment

Chemical nature and biosynthesis of oxytocin

- A peptide made of nine amino acids (a nonapeptide; *see* Figure 17.1(a))
- Molecular weight 1007 Da
- Structure similar to that of vasopressin (*see* Figure 17.1(b))
- Synthesised in *cell bodies*[1] of magnocellular neurones of the supraoptic and paraventricular hypothalamic nuclei (*see* Figure 17.2)
- Oxytocin is packaged in a secretory granule as part of a larger protein called neurophysin I
- The granule is transported down the nerve axon through the median eminence of the hypothalamus and terminates at capillaries supplying the posterior pituitary gland; oxytocin is cleaved from neurophysin 1 to release biologically active oxytocin into the circulation

---

[1] Note: vasopressin is also synthesised in cells of these brain nuclei, but mainly in the nerve terminals (*see* text).

116

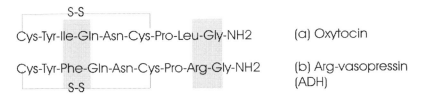

Figure 17.1 The chemical structures of (a) oxytocin; (b) arginine vasopressin (ADH). Shaded areas denote amino acid differences.

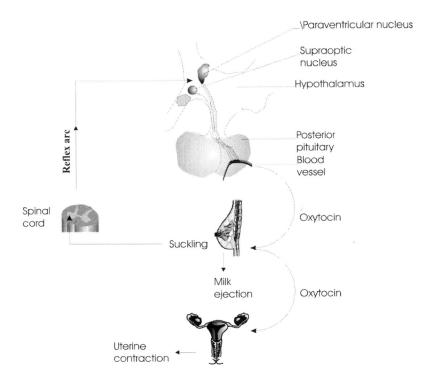

Figure 17.2 The suckling reflex.

- Some oxytocin neurones project to higher brain areas where oxytocin may mediate some aspects of sexual function and behaviour (*see* below)

Physiological actions of oxytocin

- *Stimulation of milk ejection* from the nipple (milk 'let-down') by stimulating contraction of mammary myoepithelial cells, causing milk ejection into mammary cisterns and ducts
- *Stimulation and potentiation of uterine smooth* muscle contraction during parturition (birth)
- *Promotion of maternal behaviour after* birth (but not essential for initiation or maintenance of maternal behaviour)[2]
- *Sexual behaviour:* oxytocin is possibly involved in male and female sexual behaviour and sexual arousal during copulation
- *Sperm transport:* oxytocin is possibly involved in the facilitation of sperm transport in both male and female ductal systems

Control of oxytocin biosynthesis and release and oxytocin receptor production

- *Oxytocin production* at birth is promoted by:
  - stretching of the cervix and vagina at birth
  - progesterone decline at birth.
- *Suckling reflex* (*see* Figure 17.2): oxytocin from the maternal pituitary is released by:
  - the sound of the baby crying
  - the baby's lips on the nipple and sucking.
- *Oxytocin synthesis is inhibited* by acute stress, mediated by catecholamine (epinephrine), which blocks oxytocin release from the oxytocin neurone.
- *Oxytocin receptor synthesis in the uterus* increases during late gestation due to rising secretion of estrogens.

Mechanism of action of oxytocin

- Actions of oxytocin are mediated by a membrane-associated oxytocin receptor, which is a member of the rhodopsin-type (class I group of receptors coupled to membrane G-proteins).
- The oxytocin receptor requires Mg^{2+} and cholesterol.

---

[2] From experiments with other animals.

Chemical nature, biosynthesis and secretion of vasopressin

- Also known as antidiuretic hormone (ADH)
- A peptide made of nine amino acids (a nonapeptide; *see* Fig. 17.1(b))
- Molecular weight 1084 Da
- Structure similar to that of oxytocin (*see* Figure 17.1(a))
- Synthesised in nerve endings of magnocellular neurones of the supraoptic and paraventricular hypothalamic nuclei (*see* Figure 17.2)
- Synthesised in several other brain areas
- Packaged in a secretory granule as part of a larger protein called neurophysin II
- The granule containing vasopressin is transported down the nerve axon through the median eminence of the hypothalamus and terminates at capillaries supplying the posterior pituitary gland; vasopressin is cleaved from neurophysin II to release biologically active vasopressin into the circulation
- Vasopressin neurones also project to other brain areas
- Vasopressin is also released into the pituitary stalk portal blood system (*see* p. 7), which carries it to anterior pituitary cells which secrete ACTH; vasopressin acts in concert with CRH (*see* p. 133) to regulate ACTH secretion

---

Chemical structure note: there are several different forms of vasopressin and oxytocin, depending on species, e.g. most mammals have *arginine vasopressin (AVP)*, while many non-mammals have **vasotocin**, a nonapeptide with oxytocin and vasopressin-like properties; a more primitive hormone in evolutionary terms.

Actions of vasopressin

Peripheral actions and receptors

Three distinct membrane vasopressin receptors have been identified:[3]

- V1a
- V1b
- V2

V1a mediates:

- vasoconstriction

---

[3] At the time of writing.

- platelet aggregation
- release of clotting factor VIII and von Willebrand factor
- hepatic gluconeogenesis.

V1b mediates:

- ACTH secretion from anterior pituitary corticotroph cells.

V2 mediates:

- reabsorption of water from the kidney's collecting ducts by activation of the adenylate cyclase/cyclic AMP second messenger system, which promotes insertion of aquaporin-2 channels into luminal cell membranes.

Central actions of vasopressin[4]

- Mediates aspects of social behaviour, e.g. monogamous and promiscuous animal species have different patterns of vasopressin receptor distribution in the brain
- Involved in the mediation of aggressive behaviour
- Involved in aspects of memory
- Involved in central control of temperature and blood pressure regulation

Pathophysiology of vasopressin

Diabetes insipidus

- *neurogenic (central)*: caused by hypothalamic or pituitary damage
- *nephrogenic*: caused by insensitivity of the kidneys to vasopressin; relatively rare
- *gestational*: occurs only during pregnancy.

Symptoms

- Increased urinary frequency
- Nocturia (waking at night to pass urine)
- Enuresis (bedwetting)
- Increased thirst and fluid intake
- Hypo-osmotic urine

Diagnosis

- Measurement of 24-hour urine volume
- Measurement of urine osmolality
- Serum vasopressin measurement and endocrine investigation of release
- Hypothalamic–pituitary scans

---

[4] Data include research with other species.

Treatment

- *Cranial diabetes insipidus*: administration of vasopressin analogue, e.g. desmopressin
- *Nephrogenic diabetes insipidus*:
  - paradoxical use of diuretics e.g. hydrochlorothiazide; works by promoting sodium and water excretion in the proximal tubules. Therefore less fluid is available for the distal tubules, which are affected by nephrogenic diabetes insipidus
  - balance fluid intake.

Chapter 17 quiz

Answer T (true) or F (false)

A Oxytocin:
- Is a decapeptide ☐
- Is synthesised in the hypothalamus ☐
- Stimulates milk ejection from the breast ☐
- Relaxes uterine smooth muscle ☐
- Is released from the posterior pituitary ☐
- Promotes maternal behaviour ☐
- Receptor synthesis in the uterus rises in late gestation under the influence of estrogen ☐

B Oxytocin production and release:
- Are stimulated by an increase in plasma progesterone ☐
- Are stimulated by stretching of the cervix and vagina at birth ☐
- Are stimulated by stress ☐

C Vasopressin:
- Is a nonapeptide structurally related to oxytocin ☐
- Is also called diuretic hormone ☐
- Is synthesised mainly in magnocellular neurones of hypothalamic nuclei ☐
- Is transported through neurosecretory neurones to the posterior pituitary as part of a larger protein called neurophysin II ☐

D Important actions of vasopressin include:
- Reabsorption of water from the kidney's collecting ducts ☐
- Vasodilatation ☐

E Central actions of vasopressin *may* include:
- Mediation of social and aggressive behaviour ☐
- Involvement in memory ☐
- Involvement in central control of blood pressure and temperature ☐

F Failure of vasopressin secretion results in:
- Cranial diabetes insipidus ☐
- Nephrogenic diabetes insipidus ☐
- Loss of memory ☐

G Treatment of diabetes insipidus includes:
- Balancing fluid intake ☐
- Administration of vasopressin analogues ☐
- Diuretics for nephrogenic diabetes insipidus ☐

18 The renin–angiotensin–aldosterone system

Learning objectives

- Know the three main components of the renin–angiotensin–aldosterone (RAA) system, their sources, properties, actions and termination of action
- Be able to list the three main stimuli for activation of the RAA
- Be aware of the given distinction and significance of the different angiotensin II receptor subtypes
- Be able to give some examples of drugs developed through knowledge of the RAA, and their uses

---

Definition

The renin–angiotensin–aldosterone (RAA) system is an endocrine hormone system important in the regulation of blood fluid volume and systemic blood pressure.

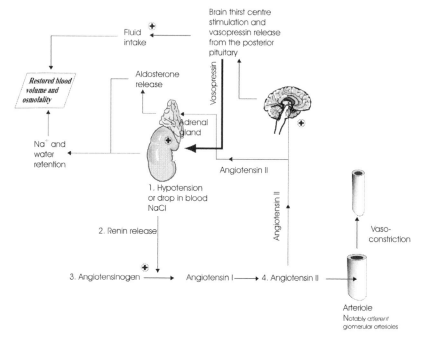

Figure 18.1 The renin–angiotensin–aldosterone system in action.

Components of the renin–angiotensin–aldosterone system (see also Figure 18.1)

Renin is an endocrine enzyme hormone secreted by the juxtaglomerular apparatus[1] of the kidney; renin is released in response to a fall in blood pressure or an abnormal rise in blood osmolality (which signals a fall in blood volume through, e.g. haemorrhage); renin catalyses the release in blood of:

- *angiotensin* (angiotensin II): a polypeptide endocrine hormone derived from a circulating blood protein angiotensinogen, which is synthesised by the liver; angiotensin II is a powerful vasoconstrictor, being particularly powerful on kidney glomerular arterioles; angiotensin also releases:
  - *aldosterone*: a steroid hormone secreted from the zona glomerulosa cells of the adrenal cortex; aldosterone acts powerfully on the distal convoluted tubules and the collecting ducts of the kidney nephron, promoting the re-uptake of Na^+ and water from the filtered urine.

---

[1] Juxtaglomerular apparatus: a group of kidney cells situated in afferent arterioles of the glomerulus. They sense blood pressure and NaCl concentration changes, and if blood perfusion pressure and NaCl fall they secrete renin.

Stimuli for activation of the renin–angiotensin–aldosterone system

- Loss in blood volume (e.g. haemorrhage)
- Loss in blood pressure caused, e.g. by haemorrhage or anaphylactic shock
- Fall in blood NaCl

Renin

- *A protein* of molecular weight $\sim$ 37 kDa
- *Alternative name:* angiotensinogenase
- *Site of biosynthesis:* juxtaglomerular cells
- *Concentration in plasma* normally $\sim$ 0.5–2.5 mg/ml
- *Stimulus for release:* fall in blood NaCl or blood volume; sympathetic nervous stimulation of α_1-and β_1 adrenoceptors on juxtaglomerular cells
- *Mechanism of action:* enzymatic cleavage of circulating angiotensinogen to *angiotensin I*, which is converted *in the lung* by angiotensin-converting enzyme $(ACE)^2$ to *angiotensin II*
- *Inactivation:* largely by the liver
- *Renin inhibitors* for treatment of hypertension are under investigation,[3] notably aliskiren (*Rasilez*® *Novartis*)

Angiotensin II

- An octapeptide
- Derived from angiotensinogen and angiotensin I in blood
- Half-life in the human circulation: $\sim$ 1–2 minutes
- *Actions:*
  - potent vasoconstrictor, especially of efferent but not afferent glomerular arterioles, resulting in increased glomerular filtration rate (*see* also below)
  - releases aldosterone from the adrenal gland
  - releases vasopressin from the posterior pituitary gland
  - direct action on proximal tubules to promote Na^+ reabsorption
  - can have prothrombic actions by aggregation and adhesion of platelets and through production of plasminogen activator inhibitor (PAI-1) and PAI-2
  - may cause hypertrophy of cardiac and vascular muscle
  - Acts on the subfornical organ[4] in the brain to stimulate thirst

---

[2] A target for antihypertensive drugs.

[3] At the time of writing.

[4] Subfornical organ: collection of osmotic Na^+ sensors close to the 3rd ventricle, beneath the fornix, responsible for generating sensation of thirst.

> *Mechanistic note*: angiotensin II constricts *efferent* glomerular arterioles preferentially, thus ensuring that the glomerulus continues to be adequately perfused in order to maintain the glomerular filtration rate.
>
> As a general rule, constriction of *afferent* arterioles feeding capillary beds results in increased arteriolar resistance, which causes a rise in blood pressure.

Angiotensin II receptors

Several subtypes have been identified:

- AT_{1A}
- AT_{1B}
- AT_2

AT$_1$ receptors

- Act via G-proteins and the inositol triphosphate (IP_3) systems
- The only angiotensin II subtype found in:
  - the aorta
  - the GIT, liver, kidney, urinary bladder, placenta

AT$_1$ and AT$_2$ receptors

- Both found in brain
- AT_2 receptors may be important in cell division and cellular proliferation

Termination of action of angiotensin II

This occurs through conversion to angiotensin III and IV by angiotensinase enzymes in the vascular beds and in red blood cells.

Drugs blocking angiotensin II action

- AT_1 receptor blockers
- Angiotensin-converting enzyme (ACE) inhibitors

AT$_1$ receptor blockers

- Reduce blood pressure by:
  - allowing vasodilation
  - reducing aldosterone production
  - reducing secretion of vasopressin
- *Uses of AT$_1$ blockers*, e.g. eprosartan (*Teveten*® *Solvay*); losartan (*Cozaar*® *MSD*):
  - treatment of hypertension

- treatment of heart failure
- in attempts to prevent or delay progression of the nephropathy of diabetes

Angiotensin-converting enzyme inhibitors

- Examples are captopril, enalapril
- Block conversion of angiotensin I to angiotensin II, and are used to treat:
  - heart failure
  - hypertension

Aldosterone

See p. 133.

The RAA system is summarised in Figure 18.1.

Chapter 18 quiz

Answer T (true) or F (false)

1 Renin is secreted by the kidney in response to a rise in blood pressure ☐

2 Renin is released also in response to a rise in blood osmolarity ☐

3 Angiotensin is derived from angiotensinogen ☐

4 Renin is an enzyme which converts angiotensin I to angiotensin II ☐

5 Angiotensin II is a powerful vasodilator in the kidneys ☐

6 Angiotensin II stimulates aldosterone release from the adrenal cortex ☐

7 Aldosterone inhibits the re-uptake of Na^+ and water in the kidney ☐

8 The RAA system is activated by haemorrhage and hypotension ☐

9 Angiotensinogen is converted to angiotensin I in the lungs ☐

A Angiotensin II:
- Is a potent selective constrictor of efferent glomerular arterioles ☐
- Stimulates vasopressin release from the pituitary ☐
- Promotes Na^+ reabsorption in the proximal tubules ☐
- Acts in the kidney through its AT_1 receptor ☐
- Action is terminatd by angiotensinase enzymes ☐

B Angiotensin AT_1 receptor blockers:
- Increase blood pressure by constricting arterioles ☐
- Reduce aldosterone production ☐
- Reduce vasopressin secretion ☐
- Are used to treat hypertension and heart failure ☐
- Are used to slow nephropathy of diabetes ☐
- Include losartan and eprosartan ☐

C ACE inhibitors:
- Block conversion of angiotensinogen to angiotensin I ☐
- Are used to treat hypertension and heart failure ☐
- Include captopril and enalapril ☐

D   Can you complete this?

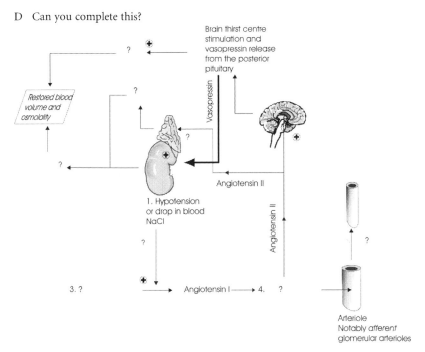

E   Can you complete this?
* A definition of the renin–angiotensin–aldosterone (RAA) system . . . . . .

19 The adrenal gland I: introduction

Learning objectives
Anatomy of the adrenal gland
Adrenocortical (adrenal cortex) hormones
Control of cortisol release from the adrenal cortex
Biosynthesis of cortisol and other adrenal steroids
Aldosterone actions and regulation of release
The adrenal medulla

Learning objectives

- Be able to make a quick sketch of the anatomical location of the adrenal glands
- Know the differences between the physiological and pharmacological actions of cortisol
- Be able to outline briefly the control of cortisol release
- Look over the biosynthetic pathways of adrenal glucocorticoid and mineralocorticoid biosynthesis
- Be able to give an account of aldosterone actions and regulation of release
- Know the hormonal actions of epinephrine

Anatomy of the adrenal gland

- *Situation*: bilaterally above the kidneys (*see* Figure 19.1(a))
- *Structure*:
  - outer adrenal cortex (*see* Figure 19.1(b))
  - inner adrenal medulla

Structure and hormones of the adrenal cortex

The adrenal cortex consists of three layers (*see* Figure 19.1(b)):

- *outer zona glomerulosa*: produces aldosterone
- *middle zona fasciculata*: thickest layer of the cortex; produces:
  - corticosteroids (also called glucocorticoids)
  - cortisol (in humans, the most powerful natural corticosteroid)
  - cortisone
  - corticosterone
  - androgens:

130

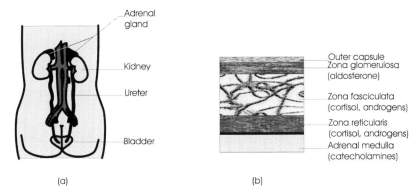

Figure 19.1 The adrenal gland. (a) Anatomical position; (b) schematic cellular layout of the adrenal cortex.

- androstenedione
- 17α-hydroxyprogesterone
- dehydroepiandrosterone sulphate (DHEAS)
- *inner zona reticularis*: surrounds the adrenal medulla; also produces androgens and corticosteroids

Structure and hormones of the adrenal medulla

- A modified ganglion, consisting of catecholamine-secreting chromaffin cells, which are modified nerve cells stained brown by chromate stains
- Releases the catecholamines *epinephrine* (adrenaline) and *norepinephrine* (noradrenaline) in response to cholinergic nervous stimulation

Adrenocortical (adrenal cortex) hormones

Cortisol is a glucocorticoid i.e. it regulates carbohydrate metabolism.

Important note: the physiological actions of cortisol, i.e. as a hormone in the body, should be distinguished from the *pharmacological* actions of glucocorticoids when administered as drugs.

Physiological actions of cortisol

Intermediary metabolism regulator

- *Anabolic action*: increases synthesis of hepatic (liver) enzymes of gluco-neogenesis
- *Catabolic action*: increases energy production in muscle and fat by breaking down the tissue and releasing free fatty acids for use as substrates for liver gluconeogenesis

Permissive actions

- Involved in the body's response to stress by allowing other hormones to act e.g. by:
  - enabling catecholamines (epinephrine and norepinephrine) to mobilise fat for energy, thus promoting maintenance of an adequate response to stress and the maintenance of a viable body temperature
  - facilitating catecholamine synthesis in the nerve terminal and its re-uptake into the nerve ending

Nervous system actions

- Role in the regulation of the body's biological 'clock'
- Regulation of hypothalamic corticotrophin-releasing hormone and anterior pituitary adrenocorticotrophin (ACTH) release by a negative feedback mechanism (*see* Fig. 19.2)
- Involved in normal brain development
- Involved in neuroprotection in adult life

Salt and water retention

- At physiological levels, mild retention by inhibiting glomerular filtration

Pharmacological actions of glucocorticoids when used for prolonged periods in high doses as drugs to treat disease

- Atrophy of the zona fasciculata and reticularis in the adrenal cortex by suppressing the release of pituitary ACTH
- Diabetes
- Gastric ulcers
- Hirsutism
- Hypertension
- Oedema
- Osteoporosis
- Psychological effects, e.g. euphoria
- Redistribution of body fat and 'moon face'
- Stunted growth in children
- Suppression of inflammatory reactions (usually the only desired effect)

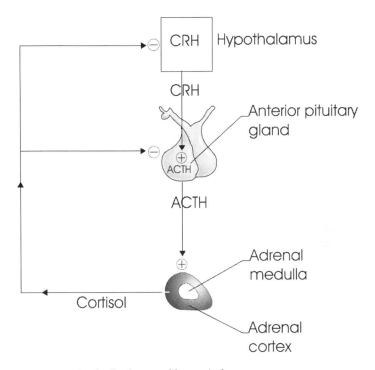

Figure 19.2 Negative feedback control by cortisol.

- Suppression of normal body responses to stress
- Suppression of the immune system and possible masking of infections
- Thinning of the skin, stretch marks and acne

Control of cortisol release from the adrenal cortex

See Figure 19.2.

Biosynthesis of cortisol and other adrenal steroids

See Figure 19.3.

Aldosterone actions and regulation of release

Actions of aldosterone

- Promotes sodium ion (Na^+) retention in the kidney, salivary and sweat glands and colon by:
  - increasing the numbers of active Na^+ channels
  - increasing the numbers of Na^+/K^+ ATPase pumps

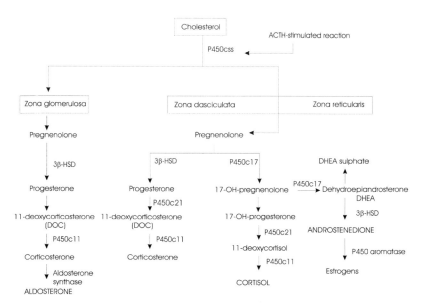

Figure 19.3 Adrenal steroid biosynthesis pathways.
Key:
    P450scc: cytochrome P450 side chain cleavage
    DHEA: dehydroepiandrosterone
    3β-HSD: 3β-hydroxysteroid dehydrogenase
    P459c11: 11β-hydroxylase
    P450c17: 17α-hydroxylase
    P450c21: 21α-hydroxylase

    – possibly promoting synthesis of subunits of the amiloride-sensitive
      channels
• Rapid non-genomic actions on Ca^{2+} mobilisation and nitric oxide production, possibly related to control of arterial vascular tone

Regulation of aldosterone release

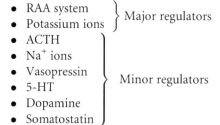

• RAA system
• Potassium ions   } Major regulators
• ACTH
• Na⁺ ions
• Vasopressin
• 5-HT   } Minor regulators
• Dopamine
• Somatostatin

The adrenal medulla

Functionally a modified sympathetic ganglion:

- innervated by cholinergic preganglionic neurones of the sympathetic nervous system
- postsynaptic medullary cells synthesise and release catecholamines norepinephrine and epinephrine, analogous to postganglionic fibres of the sympathetic nervous system

---

Embryological note: although close in anatomical terms, the adrenal cortex and adrenal medulla have different embryological origins:

- adrenal cortex from mesoderm
- adrenal medulla from the neural crest.

Structure, biosynthesis, storage and release of norepinephrine and epinephrine

- *Structure*: catecholamines, based on the catechol ring (*see* Figure 19.4)
- *Biosynthesis*: in chromaffin cell (*see* Figure 19.5(a))
- *Storage*: in vesicles
- *Release*: from the cell by cholinergic nerve impulses (*see* Figure 19.5(b))

Receptors for catecholamines

- α_1
- α_2
- β_1
- β_2
- β_3

Hormonal actions of epinephrine

Cardiovascular system

- *Heart*: increased force and rate of contraction; receptor: β_1

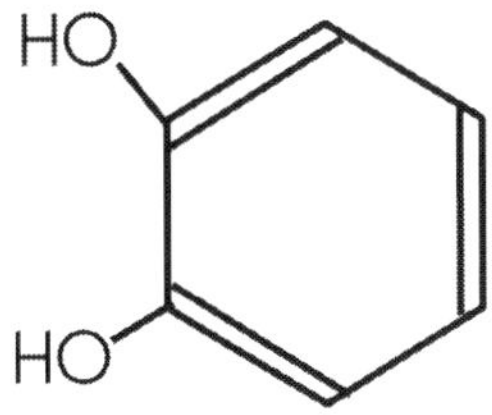

Figure 19.4 Catechol ring.

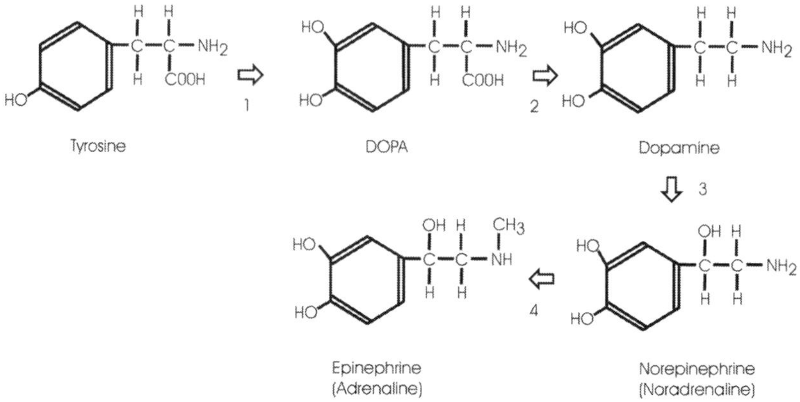

(a)

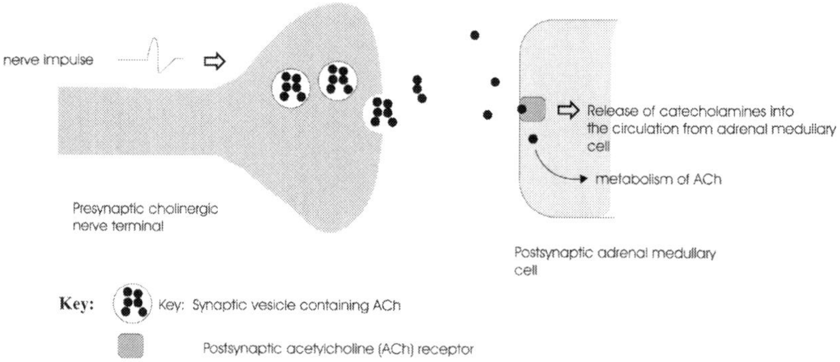

(b)

Figure 19.5 (a) Biosynthesis of catecholamines. Key to enzymes: 1, tyrosine hydroxylase: the rate-limiting reaction; 2, dopa decarboxylase; 3, dopamine β-hydroxylase; 4, phenylethanolamine *N*-methyltransferase. (b) Release of adrenal medullary catecholamines.

- *Blood vessel smooth muscle*:
  - in skeletal muscle, mucous membranes, splanchnic bed: dilate; receptor: β_2
  - in skin: constrict; receptor: α_1

Other smooth muscle
- *Bronchial tree*: bronchiolar dilatation; receptor: β_2
- *Gastrointestinal tract*:
  - smooth muscle: relaxes; receptor: α_2
  - sphincters: contract; receptor: α_1

- *Uterus, vas deferens*: contract; receptor: α_1
- *Eye*: radial muscle: contracts; receptor: α_1

Blood
- Coagulation time $\downarrow$
- Haemoglobin concentration $\uparrow$
- Plasma proteins $\uparrow$

Metabolism
- Thermogenesis (body heat generation) $\uparrow$ receptor: β_3
- Lipolysis (fat breakdown) $\uparrow$ receptor: β_3
- Glucagon release $\uparrow$ receptor: β_2
- Insulin release $\downarrow$ receptor: α_2

Chapter 19 quiz

Answer T (true) or F (false)

A   The adrenal gland:

- Is situated below the kidney
- Contains an outer cortex and inner medulla
- The outer layer of the cortex is called the zona glomerulosa
- The middle layer is called the zona fasciculata
- The inner layer is called the zona reticularis

B   Of the adrenal steroids:

- Aldosterone is synthesised mainly in the zona reticularis
- Cortisol is synthesised mainly in the zona fasciculata
- Androgens produced include androstenedione and DHEAS

C   The adrenal medulla:

- Is a modified sympathetic ganglion
- Consists chiefly of catecholamine-secreting chromaffin cells
- Releases epinephrine and norethisterone
- Releases catecholamines through cholinergic stimulation
- Surrounds the adrenal cortex

D   Cortisol:

- Is principally a glucocorticoid
- Regulates carbohydrate metabolism
- Decreases hepatic gluconeogenesis
- Promotes muscle and fat breakdown
- Inhibits catecholamine release from the nerve terminal
- Facilitates catecholamine-mediated mobilisation of fat for energy

E   Cortisol synthesis and release from the adrenal gland:

- Are inhibited by ACTH
- Are under the control of hypothalamic TRH
- Are controlled through a negative feedback action of cortisol

F   Side-effects of long-term, high doses of glucocorticoids include:

- Thinning of the skin and hirsutism
- Osteoporosis and oedema
- Exaggeration of normal body responses to stress
- Suppression of the immune system
- Gastric ulcers and hirsutism

G   Hormonal actions of epinephrine include:
- Dilatation of cutaneous (skin) arterioles through α_1 receptors
- Increased rate and force of heart contractions through β_1 receptors
- Bronchiolar tree dilatation through β_2 receptors
- Contraction of GIT smooth muscle through α_2 receptors
- Contraction of radial muscles of the eye
- Decreased coagulation time
- Increases in blood haemoglobin

H   Metabolic actions of epinephrine include:
- Increased thermogenesis
- Increased lipolysis
- Increased insulin release
- Increased glucagon release

I   Can you complete this?

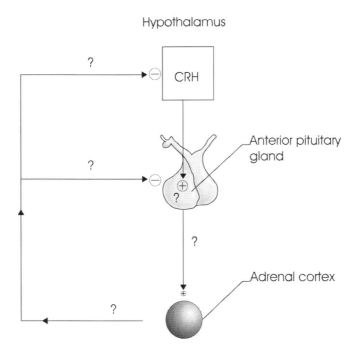

J   Can you name the structures?

Key to enzymes: 1, tyrosine hydroxylase: the rate-limiting reaction; 2, dopa decarboxylase; 3, dopamine β-hydroxylase; 4, phenylethanolamine N-methyltransferase.

20 The adrenal gland II: adrenal pathophysiology

Learning objectives
Forms of adrenocortical insufficiency (Addison's disease)
Symptoms of adrenal insufficiency
Diagnosis of adrenal insufficiency
Treatment of adrenal insufficiency
Cushing's disease and syndrome
Incidence and symptoms of Cushing's disease
Diagnosis of hypercortisolism and Cushing's disease
Treatment of Cushing's disease and syndrome

Learning objectives

- Know the distinction between Cushing's disease and the Cushing syndrome
- Understand the distinction between primary and secondary adrenal insufficiency and the symptoms
- Appreciate the principles underlying the methods used to assess the integrity of the hypothalamic–pituitary–adrenal axis in the diagnosis of hypo- and hypersecretion of cortisol
- Be able to list symptoms of the Cushing syndrome
- Be able to give an account of the approach to treatment of hypo-and hypercortisolism

Forms of adrenocortical insufficiency (Addison's disease)

Primary adrenal insufficiency

- *Cause*: damage to the adrenal cortex
- *Causative agents*:
  - TB infection
  - metastatic carcinoma
  - autoimmune attack (mostly)
  - infection, mainly fungal
- *Consequence*: reduced or absent adrenocortical steroids *including aldosterone*

Secondary adrenal insufficiency

- *Causes*:
  - pituitary damage resulting in reduced or absent ACTH secretion
  - sudden cessation of long-term glucocorticoid treatment, which has chronically suppressed ACTH secretion
- *Consequence*: reduced or absent adrenocortical steroids *except aldosterone*

Symptoms of adrenal insufficiency

Symptoms are usually of gradual onset.

- Weight loss
- Muscle weakness and fatigue
- In some patients nausea, diarrhoea and vomiting
- Hyperpigmentation (skin darkening) on various parts of the body
- Depression, irritability
- Salt craving if aldosterone secretion is impaired
- Hypoglycaemia in children
- Dysmenorrhoea or amenorrhoea
- *Addisonian crisis* (acute adrenal insufficiency if symptoms left untreated); symptoms include:
  - sudden, severe lower back pain, or pain in the lower abdomen and legs
  - diarrhoea and vomiting with consequent dehydration
  - hypotension
  - loss of consciousness
  - may be fatal if untreated

Diagnosis of adrenal insufficiency

- Skin darkening
- X-ray for calcium deposits in adrenals (symptom of TB); tuberculin test indicated if positive
- Plasma cortisol concentrations
- ACTH release test: administration of ACTH analogue and measurement of plasma/urine cortisol levels
- To test for primary adrenal insufficiency (PAI), give ACTH over 48–72 hours + measure plasma cortisol; patients with PAI have no increase in plasma cortisol during the 48–72 hours of ACTH administration
- Insulin-induced hypoglycaemia challenge (tests hypothalamic–pituitary response to stress produced by injection of quick-acting insulin): normal response – fall in blood glucose and rise in plasma cortisol within 90 minutes of insulin injection
- CT scan of pituitary gland in secondary adrenal insufficiency is diagnosed + tests of pituitary ability to release other hormones e.g. TSH, LH, FSH

Treatment of adrenal insufficiency

- Adrenal hormone replacement:
  - glucocorticoids (e.g. with hydrocortisone)
  - mineralocorticoid replacement (e.g. with fludrocortisone)
  - salt replacement if patient has primary adrenal insufficiency
- Addisonian crisis:
  - treatment for life-threatening hypoglycaemia, hypotension and hyper-kalaemia (high blood potassium): hydrocortisone, saline and dextrose IV until patient is able to take oral medication + fludrocortisone if necessary.

Clinical note: patients should be educated about dosage increases during period of stress or if suffering from upper respiratory tract infections, and about immediately reporting vomiting, diarrhoea or severe infections.

Cushing's disease and syndrome

Cushing's disease is an illness caused by overproduction of ACTH by the pituitary gland, usually because of an ACTH-secreting adenoma[1]. *Cushing's syndrome* is the appearance of the symptoms of Cushing's disease caused by:

- chronic use of glucocorticoids for other purposes, e.g. treatment of autoimmune disease (ACTH-independent; *see* Figure 20.1)
- adrenal hyperplasia, causing increased cortisol production
- benign or (very rarely) malignant cortisol-producing tumours in the adrenal gland or ectopically in e.g. lung tumours (ACTH-independent)
- alcoholism-stimulated adrenal cortisol production
- very severe depression-generated increased adrenal cortisol production.

Incidence and symptoms of Cushing's disease

- Relatively rare condition, more common in women
- Diagnosis difficult in early stages
- Muscle wasting
- Obesity centred on trunk of body
- Hirsutism
- Hypertension
- Male impotence
- Reduced libido

---

[1] A non-cancerous tumour.

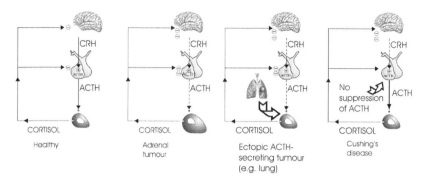

Figure 20.1 Effects of Cushing's syndrome and Cushing's disease on the hypothalamic–pituitary–adrenocortical axis.

- Rounding of the face ('moon face')
- Psychological problems, e.g. depression
- Tendency to bruising
- Abdominal stretch marks
- Diabetes mellitus
- Oligomenorrhoea[2], amenorrhoea

Diagnosis of hypercortisolism and Cushing's disease

- *24-hour urine test*: abnormally high urinary cortisol over 24 hours
- *Overnight dexamethasone test*: dexamethasone should suppress blood cortisol by inhibiting ACTH release from the pituitary gland (*see* Figure 20.1)
- *Diurnal (twice-daily) blood cortisol measurement, at 9 am and midnight*: normally, cortisol is high at 9 am and low at midnight
- *Extended dexamethasone test*: range of doses of dexamethasone four times daily over four days; distinguishes between pituitary or ectopic ACTH-producing tumour, because ectopic tumours will not usually be suppressed by high doses of dexamethasone
- *CRH test*: hypothalamic CRH normally maximally stimulates ACTH from the pituitary within 30 minutes, and cortisol from the adrenal gland within 60 minutes. In patients with ectopic ACTH secretion or cortisol-secreting adrenal tumours, there is no change in ACTH or cortisol release
- *Plasma ACTH measurement*: measurement of ACTH at 9 am will give abnormally low values due to negative feedback suppression caused by either synthetic glucocorticoids or from an adrenal cortisol-secreting tumour

---

[2] Oligomenorrhoea: irregular menses.

Other tests

- CT scans for tumours
- MRI scans for tumours

Treatment of Cushing's disease and syndrome

Treatment depends on the diagnosis.

- Surgery: transphenoidal surgery to remove a pituitary adenoma + post-operative hydrocortisone replacement
- Pituitary radiotherapy
- Adrenalectomy + lifelong hormone replacement (aldosterone is essential for life)
- Neuromodulators, e.g.:
  - GABA agonists, e.g. sodium valproate, valproic acid
  - 5-HT antagonists, e.g. cyproheptadine, ketanserin
  - dopamine agonists, e.g. bromocriptine, cabergoline
  - somatostatin analogues, e.g. octreotide

Chapter 20 quiz

Answer T (true) or F (false)

A   Primary adrenal insufficiency may be the result of damage to the adrenal cortex, caused by (e.g.):

- TB infection ☐
- Metastatic carcinoma ☐
- Autoimmune attack ☐
- Fungal infections ☐
- Pituitary damage ☐

B   Symptoms of adrenal insufficiency *may* include:

- Weight gain ☐
- Muscle weakness and fatigue ☐
- Hyperpigmentation ☐
- Addisonian crisis if untreated ☐
- Salt craving ☐
- Hyperglycaemia in children ☐
- Amenorrhoea or dysmenorrhoea ☐
- Mood depression and irritability ☐

C   Diagnosis of adrenal insufficiency includes:

- Measurement of plasma cortisol levels ☐
- ACTH-induced cortisol release test ☐
- Insulin-induced hypoglycaemia challenge ☐
- If secondary adrenal insufficiency is suspected:
  - CT scan of the pituitary ☐
  - test of pituitary ability to release other hormones, e.g. TSH ☐

D   Adrenal insufficiency is treated:

- With glucocorticoid replacement ☐
- With mineralocorticoid replacement if needed ☐
- With salt replacement for secondary adrenal insufficiency ☐
- In cases of Addisonian crisis:
  - for life-threatening hyperglycaemia ☐
  - for hypotension and hyperkalaemia ☐
  - with hydrocortisone, saline and dextrose IV ☐

E   Cushing's disease:

- Reflects under-production of ACTH by the adrenal gland ☐
- Is usually caused by an ACTH-producing adenoma ☐

F   Cushing's syndrome is the *appearance* of the disease caused by:
- Chronic use of glucocorticoids
- Adrenal hyperplasia
- ACTH-independent cortisol-producing tumours
- Increased cortisol production due to severe depression
- Alcohol insufficiency

G   Symptoms of Cushing's disease include:
- Hypotension
- Hirsutism
- Rounding of the face ('moon face')
- Male impotence
- Obesity on the trunk of the body
- Tendency to bruising
- Abdominal stretch marks
- Diabetes mellitus
- Oligomenorrhoea or amenorrhoea

H   Treatment of Cushing's disease and syndrome (depending on diagnosis) is:
- Pituitary radiotherapy
- Surgery to remove pituitary adenoma + post-operative hydrocortisone
- Adrenalectomy + permanent steroid replacement
- Neuromodulators e.g. GABA agonists, 5-HT antagonists
- Dopamine antagonists

I   Can you complete this diagram?

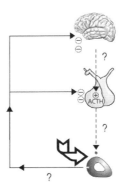

Ectopic ACTH-
secreting tumour
(e.g. lung)

21 Insulin

Learning objectives

- Know the distinction between the terms endocrine and exocrine
- Know the situation and GIT association of the pancreas in the body
- Be familiar with the different secretory cell types of the islets of Langerhans
- Be able to list the main physiological actions of insulin
- Know the inverse relationship between circulating glucose and insulin
- Be able to give a brief account of the mechanism of action of insulin
- Know the distinction between type 1 and type 2 diabetes, their aetiology, symptoms, complications and treatment

Secretions of the pancreas

- Exocrine
- Endocrine

> *Terminology note*: insulin is an *endocrine* hormone, i.e. secreted directly into the bloodstream from the hormone-producing endocrine cells of the pancreas. *Exocrine* secretions are via ducts from the glands, e.g. secretion of pancreatic digestive juices via the pancreatic duct into the duodenum.

Anatomical situation and structure of the pancreas

- Closely associated with the duodenum (*see* Figure 21.1)

148

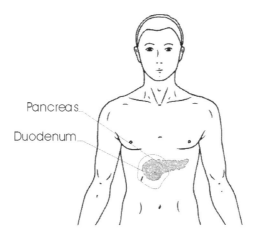

Figure 21.1 Situation of the pancreas.

- Made up mainly of exocrine grape-like clusters of *acini*, which secrete alkaline digestive juices into the duodenum via the pancreatic duct
- *The islets of Langerhans* are the *endocrine glands* of the pancreas. The islets are richly vascularised and contain several cell types:
    - α-*cells* (∼ 20% of islet cells):– secrete glucagon (*see* p. 156)
    - β-*cells* (∼ 75% of islet cells): secrete insulin
    - δ-*cells*: secrete somatostatin
    - γ-*cells*: secrete pancreatic polypeptide (function unknown)[1]

Chemical nature of insulin

- Small protein of molecular weight 6 kDa when in monomeric form
- Consists of two polypeptide chains linked through disulphide bridges (*see* Figure 21.2)

Physiological actions of insulin

- Increases uptake of amino acids and glucose from the blood into muscle, where they are converted to protein and glycogen respectively
- Acts on liver cells to:
    - stimulate glucose uptake from the blood and its conversion to glycogen
    - inhibit gluconeogenesis, i.e. breakdown of fats and proteins into glucose
    - inhibit glycygenolysis, i.e. breakdown of glycogen to glucose

[1] At the time of writing.

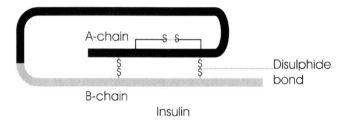

Figure 21.2 Two-chain structure of insulin.

- Acts on fat cells to:
  - stimulate glucose uptake from the blood
  - stimulate adipocytes to convert glucose to lipid stores
- Acts in the hypothalamus to suppress appetite

Therefore insulin is an *anabolic hormone*, i.e. it promotes the elaboration of polymers from simpler molecules for the storage of energy resources and for the building up of tissues, e.g. muscle.

Biosynthesis of insulin

1 Expression of insulin mRNA on the short arm of chromosome 11
2 Translation of mRNA and biosynthesis of proinsulin by the endoplasmic reticulum
3 Cleavage of proinsulin to insulin by the Golgi apparatus and in storage granules

Control of insulin release

1 Plasma glucose concentrations rise, e.g. after a meal
2 Glucose stimulates Ca^{2+} uptake by islet β-cell
3 Raised intracellular Ca^{2+} stimulates contraction of microtubules, thus moving insulin-containing storage granules to the cell membrane
4 Exocytosis occurs: the granule fuses with the cell membrane and insulin is released into the circulation
5 Insulin promotes removal of glucose from the circulation

Other insulin-releasing agents

- Other carbohydrates, amino acids, fatty acids, ketones
- Acetylcholine
- Epinephrine, acting on β-receptors (α-receptor stimulation *inhibits* insulin release)
- Glucagon

Metabolism and excretion of insulin

- Insulin half-life in plasma: ~ 5 minutes.
- Insulin monomer is filtered by glomeruli but reabsorbed in proximal tubules.
- Insulin is degraded in the kidney.
- Approximately half of all insulin secreted is removed via the hepatic portal circulation.
- Some insulin is degraded in target cells after receptor internalisation.

Mechanism of action of insulin

1 Two molecules of insulin bind to a subunit on the extracellular domain of the membrane insulin receptor.
2 Information that insulin has bound is transmitted to two transmembrane β-subunits of the insulin receptor.
3 The β-subunits autophosphorylate themselves, thus activating their built-in protein kinases.
4 This initiates an intracellular cascade of kinase protein phosphorylations and protein kinase activations, which results in the expression of action of insulin.

Insulin pathophysiology

- *Type 1 diabetes mellitus* (juvenile-onset diabetes; insulin-dependent diabetes mellitus; IDDM)
- *Type 2 diabetes mellitus* (adult-onset diabetes[2]; non-insulin-dependent diabetes mellitus; NIDDM)

Type 1 diabetes mellitus

Cause and incidence
- Presents most commonly in childhood
- Autoimmune reaction resulting in destruction of pancreatic islet β-cells, which normally secrete insulin
- Genetic abnormalities responsible for $\sim 30\%$ of cases
- Viruses and diet possibly implicated

Symptoms and consequences of failed insulin secretion
- Absence of circulating insulin
- Hyperglycaemia

---

[2] This is a dated term given the rapidly increasing incidence of juvenile obesity.

- Glucosuria (glucose in the urine)
- Polydipsia (excessive fluid intake)
- Polyuria (frequent, copious urination)
- Weight loss
- Hyperphagia (overeating)
- Microvascular complications due to hyperglycaemia, e.g. peripheral neuropathies[3] and retinopathies
- Toxic and potentially fatal build-up of circulating ketone bodies due to excessive breakdown of lipids, causing (if left untreated):
  - coma and death

Treatment
- Self-administration of insulin either orally or by injection
- Strictly controlled diet
- Regular check-ups for microvascular complications

Type 2 diabetes mellitus
Causes and incidence
- Most common form of diabetes (> 80% of cases in the UK)
- Perhaps familial in some cases
- Poor diet, obesity and sedentary lifestyle strongly implicated in aetiology
- Loss of tissue sensitivity to circulating insulin, perhaps due to:
  - decreased insulin receptors
  - decreased muscle mass, especially in sedentary patients, with consequent decreased glucose transporters across cell membranes[4]
  - reduced insulin secretion (at least in early stages)
- Poor diet and obesity, which puts great strain on the β-cells to produce insulin, leading to exhaustion of β-cells

Treatment
Important aims are:

- lower blood glucose
- treat hyperlipidaemia
- treat any hypertension
- dietary changes and weight reduction
- lifestyle changes:
  - increase physical exercise
  - stop smoking
  - cut down alcohol consumption.

---

[3] Damage to nerve endings in the extremities.
[4] Muscle is the major glucose uptake tissue.

> *Clinical note*: type 2 diabetes is associated with a greatly increased risk of death due to macrovascular accident.

Treatment of hyperglycaemia
- Dietary control and lifestyle advice (e.g. stop smoking, more exercise (*see* also above)) first, to treat hyperglycaemia, hyperlipidaemia and hypertension
- Drug treatment of hyperglycaemia:
  - *sulphonylureas* to increase insulin secretion, e.g. gliclizide, glipizide
  - metformin to enhance glucose metabolism
  - acarbose, which inhibits the enzyme α-glucosidase (keeps down plasma glucose after meals)
  - thiazolidinediones to reduce resistance to insulin, e.g. pioglitazone, rosiglitazone

Drug treatment of hyperlipidaemia
- Statins, e.g.
  - atorvastatin
  - fluvastatin
  - simvastatin

Drug treatment of hypertension
- Beta-blockers
- Diuretics

Other serious complications of diabetes
- *Peripheral neuropathies*: damage to nerve endings in extremities causing severe pain; treatments include:
  - paracetamol
  - non-steroidal anti-inflammatory drugs (NSAIDs), e.g. aspirin
  - duloxetine, amitriptyline (an antidepressant with analgesic properties)
  - gabapentin
- *Peripheral nephropathies*: damage to the kidney nephron by hypertension; treatments include:
  - diuretics, e.g. captopril, an ACE inhibitor
  - angiotensin II receptor antagonists, e.g. losartan, valsartan

Chapter 21 quiz

Answer T (true) or F (false)

1 Insulin is secreted from the islets of Langerhans ☐
2 The α-cells secrete insulin ☐
3 Insulin consists of two polypeptide chains ☐
4 The chains are connected by nucleic acid bridges ☐
5 Insulin stimulates glucose uptake into tissues from blood ☐
6 Insulin stimulates conversion of glucose to glycogen in the liver ☐
7 Insulin stimulates conversion of lipid stores to glucose in fat ☐
8 Insulin inhibits glycogenolysis, i.e. glycogen breakdown to glucose ☐
9 Insulin acts in the hypothalamus to suppress appetite ☐
10 Insulin release is stimulated by increased plasma glucose ☐
11 Glucose inhibits Ca^{2+} uptake by pancreatic islet cells ☐
12 Insulin release is blocked by raised plasma glucagon ☐
13 Insulin release is stimulated by epinephrine ☐
14 Some insulin is degraded in the kidney ☐
15 Most insulin is removed via the hepatic portal circulation ☐
16 Insulin binds to specific intracellular insulin receptors ☐
17 Insulin receptors autophosphorylate themselves ☐
18 Type 1 diabetes is insulin-dependent diabetes mellitus ☐
19 Type 2 diabetes is also called non-insulin-dependent diabetes ☐
20 Type 2 diabetes presents most commonly in childhood ☐
21 Type 1 diabetes results from autoimmune destruction of islet cells ☐
22 Treatment of type 1 diabetes mellitus is with insulin ☐
23 Type 2 (adult-onset) diabetes is associated with obesity, poor diet and a sedentary lifestyle ☐

A Failed secretion of insulin results in:

• Hyperglycaemia ☐
• Glucosuria ☐
• Polydipsia ☐
• Hyperphagia ☐
• Reduction in plasma ketone bodies ☐

B Known causes of type 2 diabetes include:

• Obesity, poor diet, sedentary lifestyle ☐
• Decreased insulin receptors ☐
• Decreased muscle mass ☐
• Reduced secretion of insulin ☐

C   Treatment aims for type 2 diabetes mellitus include:
- Increased exercise, no smoking, less alcohol
- Treat hyperlipidaemia
- Treat any hypertension
- Raise blood glucose

D   Drug treatment for hyperglycaemia employs:
- Sulphonylureas to decrease insulin secretion
- Metformin to enhance glucose metabolism
- Acarbose to reduce post-prandial glucose
- Thiazolidinediones to reduce tissue resistance to insulin
- Statins to reduce hyperlipidaemia
- Beta-blockers and diuretics to treat hypertension

E   Other serious complications of diabetes include:
- Peripheral neuropathies
- Peripheral nephropathies

F   Can you label the two structures?

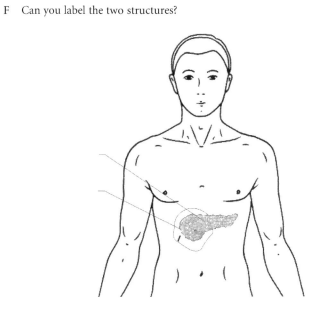

22 Glucagon

Learning objectives
Chemical nature and biosynthesis of glucagon
Control of glucagon release
Physiological actions of glucagon
Mechanism of action of glucagon
Inactivation and excretion of glucagon
Glucagon pathophysiology

Learning objectives

- Be able to give a brief outline of the nature and biosynthesis of glucagon
- Be ready to compare and contrast glucagon and insulin in terms of synthesis control and physiological actions
- Know the given symptoms of hypersecretion of glucagon

Chemical nature and biosynthesis of glucagon

- 25-amino acid polypeptide of molecular weight ~ 3.5 kDa
- Synthesised in α-cells of the islets of Langerhans; steps in biosynthesis are:
  1. expression of preproglucagon gene on chromosome 2
  2. cytoplasmic splicing of preproglucagon to yield glucagon and an N-terminal fragment called glicentin-related polypeptide fragment (GRPP)
  3. both peptides are packaged together into granules and released from the cells by exocytosis on demand

Control of glucagon release

Essentially, this is the opposite of those factors that release insulin (*see* Chapter 21):

- glucagon is released between meals when plasma fatty acids and glucose levels fall
- secretion is inhibited when energy substrates, notably plasma glucose, ketone bodies and fatty acid levels rise in plasma
- insulin inhibits glucagon release

- several GIT hormones stimulate glucagon release, e.g. cholecystokinin (CCK) and vasoactive intestinal peptide (VIP)
- the autonomic system also regulates glucagon release through both sympathetic and parasympathetic stimulation.

Physiological actions of glucagon

- Promotes hepatic (but not muscle) breakdown of glycogen to glucose
- Promotes hepatic glucose formation from amino acids
- Inhibits hepatic glycogenesis
- Stimulates free fatty acid conversion to ketone bodies
- Limited effect on lipolytic action in fat

Mechanism of action of glucagon

1 Binds to a specific glucagon receptor on the cell membrane
2 Binding activates:
   - the intracellular cyclic AMP second messenger system
   - mobilisation of intracellular Ca^{2+}
3 Glucose upregulates glucagon receptor expression
4 Glucagon and increased intracellular cyclic AMP downregulate glucagon receptor expression

Inactivation and excretion of glucagon

- Short half-life in circulation of ~ 5 minutes
- Metabolised in the liver and kidney

Glucagon pathophysiology

Glucagon-secreting tumours

- Pancreatic glucagon-secreting tumour
- *Symptoms* (some similarities to diabetes):
   - raised plasma glucose
   - weight loss
   - characteristic brown skin rash, often first appearing in groin and then spreads
   - bright red tongue
- $\sim 80\%$ of tumours are malignant, but slow-growing (survival about 15 years after diagnosis)
- *Diagnosis*:
   - measurement of circulating glucagon
   - tumour localisation

- *Treatment*:
  - surgical removal of tumour
  - chemotherapy if there is metastasis of the tumour
  - octreotide, a drug to reduce plasma glucagon
  - treatment of skin rash with IV amino acids and zinc ointment

Glucagon receptor mutations

Mutations have been discovered, particularly in patients with type 2 diabetes, especially one which results in the expression of a serine instead of a glycine residue, but the contribution of the mutation, if any, awaits elucidation.

Chapter 22 quiz

Answer T (true) or F (false)

1   Glucagon is synthesised in the α-cells of the islets of Langerhans
2   Glucagon is released when plasma fatty acids and glucose rise
3   Glucagon release is inhibited when plasma energy substrates rise
4   Insulin inhibits glucagon release
5   Glucagon is excreted mainly unchanged in the urine

A   Glucagon's actions include:
- Promotion of breakdown of glycogen to glucose in the liver
- Promotion of hepatic metabolism of amino acids to glucose
- Inhibition of hepatic glycogenesis
- Stimulation of free fatty acid conversion to ketone bodies
- A limited stimulant action on fat lipolysis

B   Glucagon's cellular actions include:
- Binding to a specific intracellular receptor
- Activation of the cyclic AMP second messenger system
- Mobilisation of intracellular Ca^{2+}
- Downregulation of its own receptor's expression

C   Glucagon over-production, e.g. by glucagon-secreting tumours:
- Produces some symptoms similar to those of diabetes
- Causes raised plasma glucose
- Causes weight loss
- Produces a brown skin rash and a bright red tongue

D   Treatment of a glucagon-secreting tumour is by:
- Surgical removal of the tumour
- Chemotherapy if the tumour is malignant
- Reduction of plasma glucagon with octreotide
- Treatment of skin rash with IV amino acids and zinc ointment

23 The thyroid gland

Learning objectives

- Know the anatomical location of the thyroid gland and its hormones
- Be able to list major actions of the thyroid hormones
- Be able to describe the steps in thyroid hormone biosynthesis and the role of TSH in biosynthesis and release of thyroid hormones from the thyroid gland
- Have knowledge of the pathways of excretion of the thyroid hormones
- Be able to list the mechanisms of action of tri-iodothyronine (T_3) and thyroxine (T_4)
- Know the types, causes, symptoms and treatment of hypo- and hyper-thyroidism

Anatomical situation of the thyroid gland

- In the neck (*see* Figure 23.1) in close proximity to the trachea
- Two lobes, each consisting of cell clusters called follicles
- Follicles are spherical, consisting of outer layers of cells surrounding a central colloid (*see* Figure 23.2)
- Contains other glandular tissue, i.e.
  - parafollicular cells: secrete calcitonin (*see* p. 191)
  - parathyroid glands: secrete parathyroid hormone (PTH)

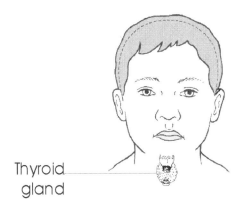

Thyroid
gland

Figure 23.1 Position of the thyroid gland in the neck.

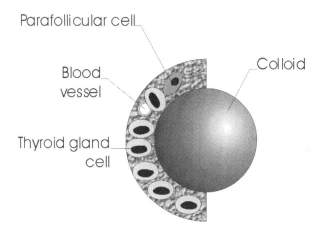

Parafollicular cell

Blood
vessel

Thyroid gland
cell

Colloid

Figure 23.2 Diagrammatic section through a thyroid follicle.

Hormones of the thyroid gland

- Thyroxine (T_4)
- Tri-iodothyronine (T_3)

Physiological actions of the thyroid hormones[1]

- Essential for normal prenatal brain and skeletal development
- Essential for proper function of growth hormone

[1] In mammals.

- Regulate the metabolic rate through:
  - mitochondrial O_2 consumption and ATP synthesis, i.e. generate energy to maintain normal body temperature (calorigenesis)
  - catabolic actions:
    - increase rate of insulin metabolism
    - stimulate GIT glucose absorption
    - stimulate adipose tissue breakdown (lipolysis)
    - stimulate liver glycogenolysis (glycogen breakdown to glucose)
    - potentiate the actions of epinephrine in breaking down glycogen to glucose (glycogenolysis)
- Reduce plasma cholesterol
- Promote vitamin A production

Biosynthesis of the thyroid hormones

Key steps in biosynthesis are:

1 iodide ion (I^-) uptake pump from blood into thyroid cells
2 oxidation of I^- to iodine (I_2) by peroxidase enzyme system
3 reaction of I_2 with tyrosine residues on thyroglobulin to form complexes of:
   - mono-iodothyronine–thyroglobulin
   - di-iodothyronine–thyroglobulin
   - tri-iodothyronine–thyroglobulin
   - thyroxine–thyroglobulin
4 which are stored in the colloid until needed.

Control of thyroid hormone release from the thyroid gland by TSH

- Thyroid-stimulating hormone (TSH) from the anterior pituitary gland controls all important steps in thyroid hormone biosynthesis and release into the circulation:
  - promotes uptake of I_2
  - promotes uptake of carbohydrates and amino acids in the thyroid cell
  - promotes thyroglobulin synthesis
  - promotes transfer of thyroglobulin from the colloid for release of free T_3 and T_4 into the thyroid cell
  - promotes release of T_3 and T_4 from the thyroid cell into the circulation
- Values for release into the circulation of thyroid hormones: T_3 and T_4: ~ 90 µg daily; T_4:T_3 ratio, ~ 20:1
- Circulating thyroid hormones are $\sim 95\%$ protein-bound, mainly to:
  - thyroxine-binding globulin (TBG)
  - thyroxine-binding pre-albumin (TBPA)
  - albumin

- Target tissue processing of thyroid hormones: T_3 is the active form of thyroid hormone, and target tissues convert most T_4 to T_3

> *Circulation note*: protein binding of hormones in blood is mainly non-covalent, and there is equilibrium between bound and free hormones; only the free hormone ($\sim 5\%$) is available to the tissues.

Metabolism and excretion of the thyroid hormones

- I^- ion released by hormone metabolism in tissues is:
  - taken back into the thyroid gland
  - excreted in the urine
  - excreted in bile after conjugation to glucuronides and sulphates in the liver
- Free thyroid hormone (a small amount) is reabsorbed through the hepatic portal system

Control of TSH release from the anterior pituitary gland

- TSH release is stimulated by hypothalamic thyrotrophin-releasing hormone (TRH; *see* Figure 23.3).[2]

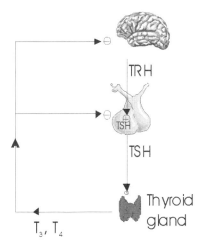

Figure 23.3 Control of thyroid hormone release.

[2] TRH also releases prolactin.

- TSH release is inhibited by T_3 through a negative feedback system.
- TSH release is therefore *increased* when circulating levels of T_4 and T_3 fall.
- TRH release is under the control of a neural pulse generator.
- TSH release is inhibited by drugs, e.g. glucocorticoids, dopamine agonists, e.g. bromocriptine.

Mechanism of action of the thyroid hormones

- Actions are mediated by cell membrane actions:
    Na^+/K^+ ATPase pump activation $\rightarrow$ increased uptake of glucose and amino acids $\rightarrow$ calorigenesis.
- Mitochondrial T_3 receptors mediate energy generation.
- Intranuclear T_3 receptors mediate transcription and *de novo* protein synthesis.

Thyroid pathophysiology

- *Hypothyroidism*: myxoedema, thyroid deficiency, autoimmune thyroiditis, Hashimoto's thyroiditis
- *Hyperthyroidism*: thyrotoxicosis, thyroid excess, Graves' disease

Hypothyroidism

Deficiency of thyroid hormones

- Primary: most common
- Central

Causes of hypothyroidism
- Iodine deficiency
- Hashimoto's autoimmune thyroiditis (most common cause)
- Iatrogenic: drugs, e.g. amiodarone, lithium, radiation or surgically induced hypothyroidism

Symptoms of hypothyroidism
- Goitre (swollen neck due to thyroid enlargement)
- Metabolism decreased, leading to:
    - anaemia
    - intolerance to cold
    - easily fatigued
    - bradycardia (heart slowing)
    - mental lethargy
    - slurred speech
    - constipation
    - hyponatraemia (lowered blood sodium)

- Brittle nails
- Dry, coarsened skin
- Joint and muscle pain

Diagnosis of hypothyroidism
- Low circulating T_3 and T_4, leading to:
  - raised circulating TSH through impaired negative feedback effect of thyroid hormones
  - raised circulating antibodies to thyroid peroxidase and to thyroglobulin (Hashimoto's thyroiditis)

Treatment of hypothyroidism
- Dietary supplements of iodine if necessary
- T_3 (lyothyronine) or T_4 (levothyroxine) orally as tablets

Cretinism
Cretinism is caused in neonates by untreated lack or severe deficiency of thyroid hormones. It is characterised by:

- mental retardation
- dwarfism
- coarsened skin and facial features.

Clinical note: early neonatal testing for hypothyroidism is very important.

Hyperthyroidism (thyrotoxicosis)
An excess of thyroid hormones caused by overactive thyroid function

- Primary: originates inside the thyroid gland
- Secondary: originates outside the gland

Causes of hyperthyroidism
Graves' disease
In older texts this is referred to as LATS (long-acting thyroid stimulator)

- Autoimmune condition, with circulating thyroid-stimulating immunoglobulin antibodies, which bind to and activate TSH receptors on thyrocytes (thyroid cells)
- More common in young women
- Symptoms include:
  - exophthalmos (Graves' ophthalmopathy) featuring protruding eyeballs

- clubbed fingers (thyroid achropachy)
- non-pitting oedema (pretibial myxoedema)[3]

Some other conditions causing hyperthyroidism
- *Toxic nodular goitre*: autonomous (unregulated) thyroid tumours, may be caused by dietary iodine deficiency
- *Subacute thyroiditis*: inflammation of the thyroid gland causing transient, abnormally high secretion of thyroid hormones
- *Toxic adenoma*: toxic multinodular adenoma

Main symptoms of hyperthyroidism
- Raised circulating T_3 and T_4
- Sweating and hyperthermia (raised body temperature)
- Sometimes exophthalmos (*see* above)
- Abnormally sensitive to heat
- Tachycardia (racing heart)
- Tremor, nervousness
- Easily fatigued
- Increased appetite coupled with weight loss

Diagnosis of hyperthyroidism
Primary
- *Low* circulating TSH
- Raised free T_4
- Raised thyroid uptake of radioactive iodide

Secondary
- *Raised* circulating TSH
- Raised free T_4
- Raised thyroid uptake of radioactive iodide

Methodology note: both total and free (unbound circulating T_3 and T_4) usually need to be measured for accurate diagnostic purposes.

Treatment of hyperthyroidism
- *Drugs*:
  - thiourylenes, e.g. carbimazole, which may work by blocking iodide $\rightarrow$ iodine conversion

---

[3] Non-pitting oedema (pretibial myxoedema): usually over the shins and does not stay depressed when pressed with the thumb.

- radioactive iodine (I^-), which destroys thyroid tissue
- aqueous iodine solution (Lugol's iodine)
- beta-blockers, e.g. propranolol, which treat symptoms e.g. tachycardia, sweating, anxiety
- *Surgery*: indicated for nodular goitres, and when the trachea is compressed

Chapter 23 quiz

Answer T (true) or F (false)

1 Primary hyperthyroidism originates outside the thyroid gland ☐
2 Secondary hyperthyroidism originates outside the thyroid gland ☐
3 Graves' disease is hyperthyroidism caused by excess iodine in water ☐

A The thyroid gland:
- Is situated behind the trachea ☐
- Consists of two lobes ☐
- Has functional units called follicles ☐
- Secretes thyroxine (T_4) and tri-iodothyronine (T_3) ☐
- Also contains parafollicular calcitonin-secreting cells ☐
- Also contains parathyroid glands which secrete thyroxine ☐

B The thyroid hormones:
- Decrease the metabolic rate ☐
- Maintain body temperature through calorigenesis ☐
- Generate energy through mitochondrial O_2 consumption ☐
- Generate energy through ATP synthesis ☐
- Are essential for the proper functioning of growth hormone ☐
- Are catabolic through:
  - decreasing the rate of insulin metabolism ☐
  - stimulation of GIT glucose absorption ☐
  - stimulation of lipolysis ☐
  - stimulation of liver glycogenolysis ☐
  - potentiation of epinephrine's stimulation of glycogenolysis ☐
- Reduce plasma cholesterol ☐
- Inhibit vitamin A production ☐

C The key steps in thyroid hormone biosynthesis are:
1 Iodide ion uptake pump from blood into thyroid cells ☐
2 Oxidation of iodide to iodine (I_2) by the peroxidase enzymes ☐
3 Reaction of I_2 with tyrosine residues on thyroglobulin ☐
4 Storage of mono-, di- and tri-iodothyronine and thyroxine in colloid ☐

D TSH controls thyroid hormone release by:
- Inhibiting the uptake of I^- into the thyroid cell ☐
- Promoting amino acid and carbohydrate uptake into thyroid cells ☐
- Blocking thyroglobulin synthesis ☐
- Promoting thyroglobulin transfer from colloid for T_3/T_4 release ☐
- Promoting T_3/T_4 release into the circulation ☐

E TSH release from the anterior pituitary:
- Is inhibited by hypothalamic TRH □
- Is inhibited by T_3 □
- Is increased when plasma levels of thyroid hormones fall □
- Is increased by high levels of glucocorticoids and dopamine agonists □

F Symptoms of hypothyroidism include:
- Goitre □
- Symptoms of lowered metabolism such as:
  - intolerance to cold □
  - easily fatigued □
  - tachycardia (rapid heartbeat) □
  - mental lethargy □
  - hyponatraemia (lowered blood sodium) □
- Brittle nails □
- Dry, coarsened skin □
- Joint and muscle pain □

G Diagnosis of hypothyroidism may include:
- Measurement of low circulating T_3 and T_4 □
- Low circulating TSH □
- Raised plasma antibodies to thyroid peroxidase and thyroglobulin □

H Treatment of hypothyroidism involves:
- T_3 or T_4 □
- Dietary iodine supplements if necessary □

I Symptoms of Graves' disease include:
- Exophthalmos (protruding eyeballs) □
- Clubbed fingers □
- Non-pitting oedema □

J The main symptoms of hyperthyroidism may include:
- Raised circulating T_3 and T_4 □
- Hyperthermia and sweating □
- Exophthalmos □
- Nervousness and tremor □
- Easily fatigued □
- Increased appetite coupled with weight loss □
- Abnormal sensitivity to cold □

K Treatment of thyrotoxicosis involves drugs, including:
- Thiourylenes, e.g. carbimazole □

- Radioactive iodine ☐
- Aqueous iodine solution ☐
- α_1-blockers ☐

24 Endocrine hypertension

Learning objectives
Hypertension
Properties of hypertension
Endocrine hormones and conditions often associated
    with endocrine hypertension
Liddle syndrome

Learning objectives

- Know the given definition and properties of hypertension
- Be able to list the endocrine-related conditions associated with hypertension
- Be able to mention briefly how the hormones mentioned here may be implicated in endocrine hypertension

Hypertension

Essential hypertension

- No known cause[1]; not dealt with here
- Currently incurable, although can be treated with antihypertensive drugs

Endocrine hypertension

- Hypertension usually due to inappropriate endocrine hormone release into the bloodstream
- Often curable

Properties of hypertension

- Systolic blood pressure consistently more than 140 mmHg (mm mercury)
- More importantly: diastolic blood pressure more than 90 mmHg
- Risks with chronic hypertension, essential or endocrine:
  - renal (kidney) failure
  - stroke
  - myocardial infarction (heart attacks)
  - heart failure

---

[1] At the time of writing.

Clinical note: diastolic blood pressure measures the total peripheral resistance (TPR), i.e. no contribution from the heart; TPR will be raised due to increased resistance from the peripheral vascular beds due to constriction of arterioles and/or obstructions to blood flow. Healthy people can have raised systolic pressure, e.g. during exercise or stress. Therefore diastolic blood pressure is a more reliable indicator of chronic hypertension.

Endocrine hormones and conditions often associated with endocrine hypertension

Adrenal and related disorders[2]

Congenital adrenal hyperplasia

This is a cluster of inherited disorders affecting the adrenal glands, caused by deletion of enzymes necessary for cortisol and aldosterone production, resulting in overproduction of androgens and of deoxycorticosterone (DOC), which has aldosterone-like activity and causes excess Na^+ retention and hypertension. Treatment is with synthetic glucocorticoids.

Cushing's disease

In Cushing's disease with glucocorticoid excess (*see* also p. 141), excess circulating cortisol promotes excessive angiotensinogen production in the liver and over-activity of angiotensin II, resulting in excessive Na^+ retention and hypertension. Treatment is usually surgical:

- to remove sources of glucocorticoid-releasing tumours
- to remove pituitary ACTH-secreting tumours
- if surgery is not possible, with drugs to reduce glucocorticoid production, e.g. ketoconazole, aminoglutethimide.

Phaeochromocytoma (catecholamine-secreting tumour)

This is a catecholamine-producing tumour in the adrenal medulla or ectopically[3] in the body. Symptoms during an attack reflect over-activity of epinephrine and include:

- sweating
- racing heart (palpitations)
- tremor

[2] This list is not comprehensive.
[3] Ectopic: abnormal anatomical location.

- headache
- anxiety
- dispnoea
- pallor.

Treatment is surgical removal of the tumour.

Surgical note: patients are given α-adrenergic-blocking drugs pre-operatively because physical handling of the tumour can cause dangerous release of epinephrine.

Primary hyperaldosteronism

In primary hyperaldosteronism with excess mineralocorticoid excretion, there is abnormally high secretion of aldosterone, usually due to aldosterone-secreting adrenal adenomas; treatment is removal of the tumour; in a small number of cases the cause is unknown and aldosterone receptor antagonists, e.g. spironolactone, are prescribed.

Thyroid disorders

Hyperthyroidism

Hyperthyroidism causes hypertension through effects on the heart (increased cardiac output) and through a lowering of the TPR.

Hypothyroidism

Hypothyroidism causes diastolic hypertension through increased circulating cholesterol and increased plasma fatty acids.

Diabetes mellitus

- Causes hypertension associated with obesity, insulin resistance and hyper-insulinaemia, which all interfere with proper glucose uptake by tissues, resulting in abnormally high circulating insulin
- Insulin both promotes Na^+ reabsorption in the nephron and enhances sympathetic drive to the heart and blood vessels, which may cause hypertension

Renal disorders

- Hypertension can damage kidneys, making hypertension worse.
- Kidney disease, e.g. renal tumours, with impairment of the renin–angiotensin regulatory system can cause abnormal circulating Na^+, with resultant hypertension.

Sex hormones and sexual function

- Hypertension of pregnancy:
  - pregnancy can induce hypertension, which usually develops after 20 weeks' gestation. It may be familial or an estrogen-induced effect
  - pre-eclampsia is hypertension of pregnancy in a previously normotensive woman.
- Hypertension associated with estrogen use, e.g. estrogen-containing oral contraceptives, HRT.

Liddle syndrome

This is an autosomal dominant inheritance of hypertension, usually early-onset, with abnormally low aldosterone secretion.

Chapter 24 quiz

Answer T (true) or F (false)

1 Endocrine hypertension has no known cause ☐

2 Endocrine hypertension is often curable ☐

3 Either hyperthyroidism or hypothyroidism could cause hypertension ☐

4 Diabetes mellitus can cause hypertension ☐

5 Over-activity of the RAA system can cause hypertension ☐

6 Pregnancy provides protection against hypertension ☐

A Risks with chronic hypertension include:
- Stroke ☐
- Myocardial infarction ☐
- Heart failure ☐
- Kidney failure ☐

B Endocrine disorders often associated with endocrine hypertension include:
- Congenital adrenal hyperplasia ☐
- Disorders of glucocorticoid deficiency ☐
- Phaeochromocytoma ☐
- Primary hyperaldosteronism with excess mineralocorticoid secretion ☐

25 Appetite regulation and obesity

Learning objectives
Regulation of appetite
Obesity
'Metabolic syndrome'

Learning objectives

- Know the given roles of adipose tissue and the nature, role and actions of leptin and aponectin
- Be able to list some suggested causes of obesity and high-risk factors associated with obesity
- Be aware of the term 'metabolic syndrome' and of its endocrine components

Regulation of appetite

- Peripheral components:
    - adipose tissue and adipose tissue hormones
- Central (brain) components:[1]
    - hypothalamus and higher centres

Peripheral components

Adipose tissue
- *Composition*: made up of adipocyte cells filled with triglycerides
- *Metabolic role*:
    - energy storage: source of free fatty acids
    - insulation
    - degree of insulin resistance
- *Endocrine role*: hormone production, notably:[2]
    - leptin
    - adiponectin
    - resistin
    - TNF-α
- *Cardiovascular role*:
    - releases plasminogen activator inhibitor (PAI-1)

---

[1] Evidence is mainly from other species, e.g. mice, rats.
[2] Not comprehensive; others, e.g. angiotensin, estradiol, IL-6 also detected.

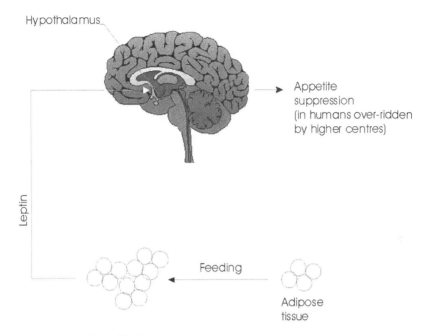

Hypothalamus

Appetite
suppression
(in humans over-ridden
by higher centres)

Leptin

Feeding

Adipose
tissue

Figure 25.1 Action of leptin.

Leptin

- *Main source*: adipose tissue
- *Chemical nature*: protein hormone, molecular weight ~ 16 kDa
- *Role*: regulation of appetite and energy homeostasis (*see* Figure 25.1); satiety hormone

Central components

Hypothalamus and higher centres

- *Site of action of leptin*: hypothalamus
- *Mechanism of action*: leptin receptors – several subtypes
- *Effects*:
  - inhibits hypothalamic activity of hypothalamic neurons that express the potent appetite stimulants:
    - agouti-related peptide
    - neuropeptide Y
  - increases hypothalamic activity of hypothalamic nuclei that express α-melanocyte-stimulating hormone (α-MSH), a peptide which mediates satiety

   – downregulates expression of endocannabinoids, which are appetite
     stimulants
   – stimulates angiogenesis[3] in endothelial cells
   – possible role in human obesity, because mutant leptin receptors occur
     in a rare form of obesity characterised by obsessive eating

Adiponectin
- *Main source*: adipose tissue
- *Chemical nature*: polypeptide (244 amino acids)
- *Roles*:
   – increases tissue sensitivity to insulin, therefore protects against type 2
     diabetes
   – has anti-inflammatory properties
   – promotes weight reduction by:
      – triglyceride clearance
      – glucose uptake into adipose tissue
      – suppression of glycogenolysis in liver
      – increasing free fatty acid uptake from the circulation into muscle
   – protects the endothelium of blood vessels from plaque formation

Obesity
Definitions of obesity (several available)
- Overweight by 30% or more of ideal body weight[4]
- Body mass index (BMI)[5] more than 30
- Waist:hip ratio 1 or more[6]

Some suggested causes of obesity
- Dietary excess and overindulgence in high-calorie foods and alcohol
- Sedentary lifestyle and lack of exercise
- Poor dietary education
- Poverty
- Mental illness, e.g. stress, depression
- Metabolic disorders
- Possible ethnic factors
- Perhaps genetic factors (very little evidence as yet)

---

[3] Angiogenesis: development of new blood vessels.
[4] Ideal body weight charts take into account sex and age.
[5] BMI: a person's weight in kg divided by (height in m)^2 (BMI = kg/m^2).
[6] Ratio of waist:hip circumference.

High-risk factors associated with obesity

- Coronary heart disease
- Excessive perspiration
- Heart failure
- Thromboembolism
- Insulin resistance and type 2 diabetes
- Hirsutism in women
- Hypertension
- Hyperlipidaemia
- Infertility
- Kidney disease
- Respiratory disorders
- Physical disability and mobility restriction
- Osteoarthritis
- Stroke
- Vascular problems, e.g. varicose veins
- Cancer (particularly in women):
  - breast
  - kidney
  - colon
- Premature death from:
  - cancer
  - cardiovascular disease

'Metabolic syndrome'

Cluster of metabolic disorders in one patient

- endocrine components:
  - glucose intolerance
  - hyperinsulinaemia and insulin resistance
  - hypercortisolism
  - hypertriglyceridaemia
  - raised LDL and lowered HDL

Chapter 25 quiz

Answer T (true) or F (false)

1   The main source of leptin is the hypothalamus

2   Leptin stimulates appetite

3   Leptin's site of action for suppressing appetite is the hypothalamus

4   Leptin downregulates hypothalamic endocannabinoid[7] expression

5   Leptin stimulates angiogenesis[8] in endothelial cells

A   Leptin inhibits the activity of neurones which express:

- Neuropeptide Y
- Agouti-related peptide
- α-MSH

B   Adiponectin:

- Is a hormone secreted by adipose cells
- Decreases tissue sensitivity to insulin
- Promotes triglyceride clearance
- Promotes glucose uptake into adipose tissue
- Suppresses glycogenolysis in liver
- Increases fatty acid uptake from blood into muscle
- Protects blood vessel endothelium from plaque formation

C   High-risk factors associated with obesity include:

- Hypotension
- Breast cancer
- Coronary heart disease
- Type 2 diabetes mellitus and insulin resistance
- Heart failure
- Hypolipidaemia
- Kidney problems
- Baldness
- Mobility problems
- Osteoarthritis
- Stroke

D   Endocrine components of the 'metabolic syndrome' include:

- Hypocortisolism

[7] Endocannabinoids are appetite stimulants.

[8] Angiogenesis is the formation of new blood vessels.

- Glucose intolerance ☐
- Insulin resistance and hyperinsulinaemia ☐
- Hypertriglyceridaemia ☐
- Raised LDL and lowered HDL ☐

26 Parathyroid hormone and parathyroid hormone-related protein

Learning objectives
Parathyroid hormone
How increased Ca^{2+} in plasma is achieved by
  parathyroid hormone
Control of parathyroid hormone release
Effects of parathyroid hormone on bone
Mechanism of action of parathyroid hormones
Parathyroid hormone pathophysiology
Parathyroid hormone-related protein
The extracellular calcium-sensing receptor

Learning objectives

- Know the anatomical location of the parathyroid glands
- Know briefly how parathyroid hormone (PTH) increases Ca^{2+} in plasma, and the effects of PTH on bone
- Be able to give a brief account of the control of PTH release
- Be aware of the existence of the two known types of PTH receptor and of their binding selectivity
- Know the given classification and causes of the three forms of hyperparathyroidism, and be aware that symptoms are similar to those of hypercalcaemia
- Be aware of the existence of parathyroid hormone-related protein (PTHrP) and of the extracellular calcium-sensing receptor

Parathyroid hormone

- Secreted from parathyroid glands embedded in the thyroid gland (*see* Figure 26.1)
- *Chemical nature*: a linear protein of 84 amino acids, cleaved from a 90-amino acid precursor called pro-PTH
- *Functions*:
  - to increase calcium ion (Ca^{2+}) concentrations in blood
  - to decrease phosphate ion concentrations in blood

182

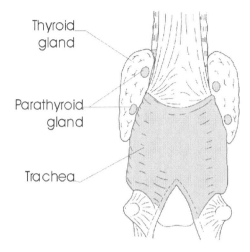

Thyroid gland

Parathyroid gland

Trachea

Figure 26.1 Anatomical location of the parathyroid glands.

- *Receptor types*:
  - type I parathyroid hormone receptor binds both PTH and PTHrP
  - type 2 parathyroid hormone receptor binds PTH selectively

How increased Ca^{2+} in plasma is achieved by parathyroid hormone (see Figure 26.2)

- Increase of Ca^{2+} absorption in the GIT indirectly by stimulating production of active vitamin D in the kidney
- Mobilisation of Ca^{2+} from bone by stimulating osteoclasts to resorb bone
- Reduction of Ca^{2+} loss in urine by enhancing tubular reabsorption of Ca^{2+}

Control of parathyroid hormone release

- PTH release from the parathyroids is increased by low plasma and other extracellular concentrations of Ca^{2+}.
- The parathyroid gland detects low extracellular Ca^{2+} by means of a *calcium-sensing receptor* on the parathyroid cell surface; the receptor is also expressed on cell membranes of C cells of the thyroid gland.

Effects of parathyroid hormone on bone

- Fast (within minutes) release of Ca^{2+} from bone
- Periods of prolonged PTH plasma levels cause:
  - bone remodelling
  - increased bone resorption by osteclasts

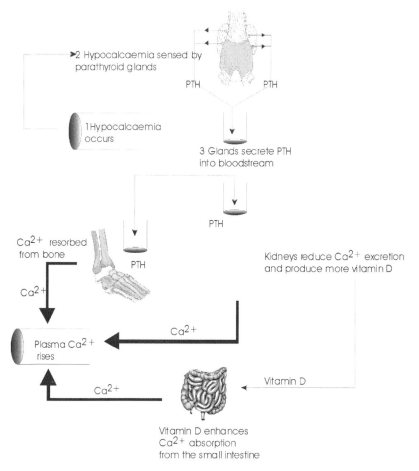

Figure 26.2 How Ca^{2+} concentration in plasma is increased by parathyroid hormone.

Mechanism of action of parathyroid hormones

Type 1 PTH receptor

- Binds both PTH and PTHrP (*see* below)
- G-protein-coupled membrane receptor
- Binding activates cyclic AMP and inositol triphosphate (IP_3) second messenger systems
- Expressed mainly in bone, but also at lower levels in many other tissues

Type 2 PTH receptor

- Binds PTH selectively
- Expressed in relatively few tissues
- Binding activates cyclic AMP system
- Poorly understood

Parathyroid hormone pathophysiology

Hyperparathyroidism

Primary hyperparathyroidism

- Hypercalcaemia caused by over-secretion of PTH from the parathyroid glands
- Cause is usually a benign PTH-secreting adenoma in the parathyroid gland; rarely caused by a parathyroid gland carcinoma
- More common in women

Symptoms of hyperparathyroidism

Symptoms of primary hyperparathyroidism are similar to those of hypercalcaemia:

- *effects on bone*:
  - osteomalacia: bone softening
  - osteoporosis: loss of bony tissue causing fragile, easily fractured bone
  - arthritis
  - osteitis fibrosa cystica: osteitis is inflammation of bone
- *effects of hypercalcaemia on the GIT*:
  - acute pancreatitis
  - constipation
  - nausea and vomiting
  - indigestion
  - peptic ulceration
- *effects of hypercalcaemia on the CNS*:
  - ataxia (unsteady walking, difficulty with balance)
  - coma
  - delirium
  - depression
  - energy loss (fatigue)
  - memory loss
  - physical weakness
  - psychosis.

Diagnosis of primary hyperparathyroidism

- Measurement of serum Ca^{2+}: abnormally raised
- Measurement of serum PTH: abnormally raised

Treatment of primary hyperparathyroidism
- Usually surgery to remove the adenoma

Secondary hyperparathyroidism
- Usually secondary to renal failure, when kidneys:
  - fail to synthesise active vitamin D
  - fail to excrete phosphate adequately, which promotes insoluble calcium phosphate formation, which removes Ca^{2+} from the circulation

---

Feedback note: the parathyroids respond to lowered circulating Ca^{2+} by releasing more and more PTH.

- Secondary to vitamin D dietary deficiency:
  - active vitamin D suppresses expression of PTH by inhibiting transcription of PTH mRNA
  - vitamin D deficiency reduces efficiency of Ca^{2+} reabsorption from the kidney tubule, leading to excessive PTH production
- GIT malabsorption problems
- Often asymptomatic

Treatment of secondary hyperparathyroidism
- Vitamin D replacement
- Phosphate-binding agents

Tertiary hyperparathyroidism
- Tertiary hyperparathyroidism results from establishment of autonomous parathyroid gland activity disconnected from circulating PTH levels, or perhaps from resetting of the feedback effect of Ca^{2+} ions.
- It is usually the consequence of a very long period of secondary hyperparathyroidism and chronic renal disease.
- Diagnosis is possibly made on the basis of inability to treat hypercalcaemia and inability to treat osteomalacia with vitamin D therapy.

Parathyroid hormone-related protein
What is it?
- A protein hormone produced by virtually all the tissues in the body

What is its nature?
- Many forms exist, depending on the tissue expressing it; one gene expresses it, but the nature of the hormone depends on the tissue-specific splicing of the mRNA produced.

Physiological effects of parathyroid hormone-related protein

- Many effects of PTHrP are unrelated to PTH action; many are paracrine and autocrine actions. The list is not comprehensive.
- Some examples of PTHrP action are:
  - control of cellular differentiation, proliferation and cell death
  - important role in tissue and organ development
  - some effects on Ca^{2+} fluxes in tissues
  - possible role in maintenance of hair follicle function
  - possible role in maternal–fetal Ca^{2+} transfer
  - smooth muscle relaxant
  - eruption of developed teeth from gums.

The extracellular calcium-sensing receptor

What is it?

- A receptor originally discovered on the surface of parathyroid cells, which binds Ca^{2+} ions. It has been detected also on cells of e.g. kidney, bone marrow haematopoietic cells and GIT mucosa.

What are its intracellular second messengers?

- Activation of the receptor by Ca^{2+} activates the IP_3 system and inhibits the cyclic AMP system

What is its clinical significance?

- Mutations of the receptor have been discovered in humans who suffer from calcium resistance, e.g. familial hypocalciuric hypercalcaemia
- *Conclusion*: Ca^{2+} is an endocrine hormone which controls or regulates its own homeostasis

Chapter 26 quiz

Answer T (true) or F (false)

A   The parathyroid glands:
- Are situated below the thyroid gland ☐
- Secrete parathyroid hormone (PTH) ☐

B   Parathyroid hormone:
- Decreases Ca^{2+} concentrations in the blood ☐
- Decreases PO_4^{3-} concentrations in the blood ☐
- Increases plasma Ca^{2+} by:
    - stimulating kidney production of vitamin D ☐
    - mobilisation of Ca^{2+} from bone ☐
    - enhancing tubular re-absorption of Ca^{2+} ☐

C   PTH release:
- Is decreased by low extracellular Ca^{2+} concentrations ☐
- Is partly controlled by a Ca^{2+} sensor receptor on the parathyroid cell ☐

D   PTH effects on bone:
- Are relatively slow ☐
- Include bone remodelling ☐
- Result in bone resorption by osteoclasts ☐

E   The mechanism of action of PTH:
- Is through membrane-bound type I/type II PTH receptors ☐
- Is also through:
    - type I PTH receptors are G-protein coupled and activate both cyclic AMP and IP_3 second messenger systems ☐
    - type I PTH receptors are expressed poorly in bone ☐

F   In primary hyperparathyroidism:
- Hypercalcaemia is caused by under-secretion of PTH ☐
- The cause is usually a malignant PTH-secreting adenoma ☐
- The disorder is more common in women ☐

G   Symptoms of primary hyperparathyroidism:
- Are similar to those of hypercalcaemia ☐
- Include:
    - bone softening (osteomalacia) ☐
    - osteoporosis ☐
    - arthritis ☐
    - osteitis fibrosa cystica (inflammation of bone) ☐

H   Effects of hypercalcaemia on the gastrointestinal tract include:
- Acute pancreatitis
- Diarrhoea
- Nausea and vomiting
- Peptic ulceration

I   Effects of hypercalcaemia on the central nervous system include:
- Ataxia, unsteady gait; difficulty with balance
- Hyperactivity
- Coma
- Delirium
- Depression
- Memory loss
- Psychosis (loss of contact with reality)

J   Secondary hyperparathyroidism is usually secondary to renal failure, when the kidneys:
- Over-secrete active vitamin D
- Fail to secrete phosphate adequately

K   Tertiary hyperparathyroidism:
- May result from:
    - establishment of autonomous PTH gland activity disconnected from circulating PTH levels
    - resetting of the Ca^{2+} effect on bone
- Is possibly diagnosed on the basis of an inability to treat hypercalcaemia and osteomalacia with vitamin D therapy

L   Parathyroid-hormone-related protein (PTHrP):
- Is produced only by parathyroid cells
- Exists in several forms
- Binds to both the type I PTH and PTHrP receptors
- Has many actions, including:
    - control over cellular differentiation, proliferation and cell death
    - relaxing smooth muscle

M   Can you complete this diagram?

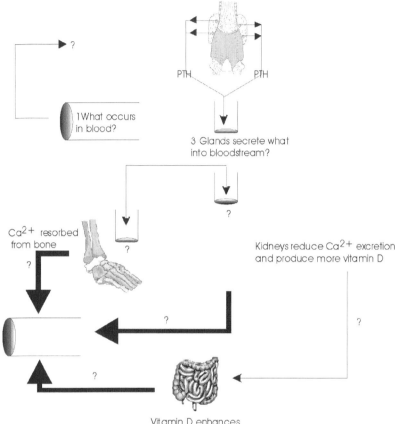

27 Calcitonin

Learning objectives
Source, synthesis and nature of calcitonin
Actions of calcitonin
Mechanism of action of calcitonin
Clinical uses of calcitonin

Learning objectives

- Know the source of calcitonin secretion
- Be aware of the existence of procalcitonin, a precursor of calcitonin
- Be able to list the known actions of calcitonin, especially its effects on Ca^{2+}
- Know that the calcitonin receptor is membrane bound and linked to the cyclic AMP system
- Be able to list the present clinical uses of calcitonin

Source, synthesis and nature of calcitonin

- *Source*: C (clear) cells in the human thyroid gland
- *Nature*: a 32-amino acid polypeptide
- *Biosynthesis*:
  - mRNA for the precursor procalcitonin in expressed by the *CALCI* gene on the short arm of chromosome 11 (*see* Figure 27.1)
  - procalcitonin is cleaved by proteolytic enzymes to yield calcitonin
  - procalcitonin is detected in plasma in the presence of severe sepsis associated with infection
  - calcitonin is secreted from the C cell
  - mRNA expressed by the *CALCI* gene can be spliced alternatively to yield another polypeptide called *calcitonin gene-related peptide*, possibly involved in vascular and nervous function, apparently unrelated to Ca^{2+} control

Actions of calcitonin

In humans, calcitonin is not as important in Ca^{2+} regulation as is PTH.

- Reduces blood calcium by:
  - reducing bone osteoclast activity, thus protecting bone from demineralisation
  - reducing Ca^{2+} absorption from the GIT
  - reducing Ca^{2+} (with accompanying phosphate) reabsorption from the tubules of the kidneys

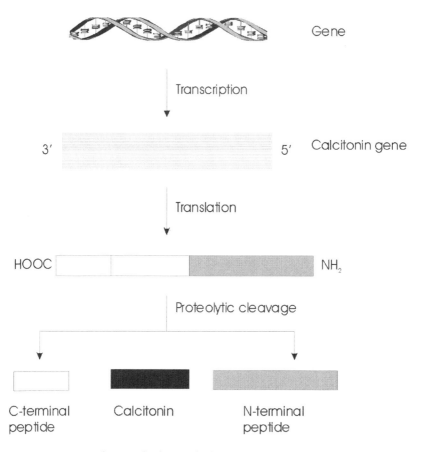

Figure 27.1 Biosynthesis and splicing of calcitonin gene products.

- Indirectly promotes vitamin D production by reducing plasma Ca^{2+}; this promotes PTH release, which in turn promotes vitamin D synthesis by the kidney
- May be a satiety hormone (like leptin); inhibits feeding, possibly by a direct action in brain (this also reduces prandial Ca^{2+} intake)
- May protect the body from bone loss during pregnancy and stress

Mechanism of action of calcitonin

- Acts through a membrane receptor linked to the cyclic AMP second messenger system
- Calcitonin and PTH receptors have similarities in amino acid sequence

Clinical uses of calcitonin

Calcitonin is now largely displaced by the bisphosphonates, but is still listed in the *BNF*.

- Prescribed as salmon calcitonin
- *Uses*:
  - metastases of bone
  - postmenopausal osteoporosis
  - Paget's disease of bone (*see* p. 199)
  - hypercalcaemia
  - to protect against bone loss during illness and immobility

Chapter 27 quiz

Answer T (true) or F (false)

1   Calcitonin is synthesised in clear (C) cells in the thyroid gland

2   Calcitonin is a lipoprotein hormone

3   Calcitonin is derived from a precursor called procalcitonin

4   Calcium acts through an intracellular receptor linked to the cyclic AMP system

A   Calcitonin's actions include:
- Reduction of blood calcium by:
    - increasing bone osteoclast activity
    - reducing Ca^{2+} absorption from the GIT
    - reducing Ca^{2+} reabsorption from the kidney tubules
- Promotion of vitamin D production
- Possibly acting as a satiety hormone, reducing dietary Ca^{2+} intake

B   Uses of calcitonin (prescribed as salmon calcitonin) include:
- Treatment of bone metastases
- Treatment of postmenopausal osteoporosis
- Hypocalcaemia
- Protection against bone loss during illness and immobility

28 Vitamin D (cholecalciferol and ergocalciferol)

Learning objectives
Nature of vitamin D
Production and activation of vitamin D (in humans)
Some food sources of vitamin D
Physiological actions of vitamin D
Control of vitamin D synthesis
Mechanism of action of vitamin D
Causes of vitamin D_3 deficiency
Symptoms of vitamin D_3 deficiency
Clinical use of vitamin D
Adverse effects of vitamin D

Learning objectives

- Know the names of the different forms of vitamin D and their biosynthesis
- Be able to give an account of the production and activation of vitamin D
- Be able to list the physiological actions of vitamin D
- Know that vitamin D production is regulated by parathyroid hormone (PTH)
- Know that vitamin D's effects are mediated by an intracellular receptor
- Be able to list some causes and symptoms of vitamin D deficiency and know that treatment is with oral vitamin D supplements

Nature of vitamin D

- Combination of several compounds which are different forms of calciferol
- The active form is 1,25-dihydroxyvitamin D_3 (1,25-$(OH)_2$-D_3; also called calcitriol)

Production and activation of vitamin D (in humans)

See Figure 28.1.

1 Sunlight stimulates conversion of 7-dehydrocholesterol to cholecalciferol (vitamin D_3)
2 Cholecalciferol is then converted in the liver to 25-hydroxycholecalciferol (25-hydroxyvitamin D_3)

195

3   25-hydroxycholecalciferol is then converted in the kidney to the biologically active 1,25-dihydroxycholecalciferol (1,25-dihydroxyvitamin D_3)
through the action of parathyroid hormone (PTH)

Some food sources of vitamin D

- Milk (especially when fortified with vitamin D)
- Fish liver oils, e.g. cod liver oil
- Eggs

Physiological actions of vitamin D (see Figure 28.1)

- Promotion of calcium absorption from the GIT
- Stimulation of calcium resorption from bone
- Stimulation of proteins involved in Ca^{2+} transport across GIT membrane
- Possibly stimulates Ca^{2+} reabsorption and phosphate excretion in the kidneys
- May be important in maturation of haematopoietic stem cells

Control of vitamin D synthesis

- PTH is the major regulator of vitamin D production in the kidney.

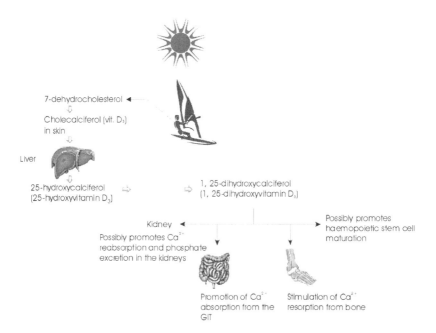

Figure 28.1 Vitamin D activation and actions.

Mechanism of action of vitamin D

- Similar to that of other lipophilic hormones, e.g. the steroid hormones
- Fat-soluble vitamin D penetrates easily through the cell membrane and binds to a cytoplasmic receptor
- The complex passes to the nucleus where it alters gene expression

Causes of vitamin D_3 deficiency (not comprehensive)

- Dietary deficiencies
- Clothing that bars sunlight
- Ageing
- Chronic diseases, e.g.
  - cancer
  - diabetes
  - hypertension
  - inflammatory bowel disease
  - kidney damage
  - liver cirrhosis
  - mutations of the vitamin D_3 receptor
  - rheumatoid arthritis

Symptoms of vitamin D_3 deficiency

- Rickets in children, with symptoms of bone weakness, e.g. bowed long bones
- Osteomalacia in adults, with bone thinning and symptoms of bone pain, muscle weakness and numbness around the mouth (symptom of calcium deficiency)
- Osteoporosis, bone porosity and consequent fragility

Clinical use of vitamin D

- The *BNF* states that simple vitamin D deficiency can be prevented by taking an oral supplement of 10 µg ergocalciferol daily
- 'Vitamin D' covers the use of:
  - cholecalciferol (D_3)
  - ergocalciferol (D_2)
  - calcitriol (1,25-dihydroxycholecalciferol)

Adverse effects of vitamin D

- Vitamin D is not generally considered toxic, and toxicity is more usually due to overdoses of vitamin A in e.g. liver oils.
- Overdosage of vitamin D has been reported (rarely) to cause hyper-calcaemia and atherosclerosis, which may be fatal.

Chapter 28 quiz

Answer T (true) or F (false)

1 Vitamin D is a collective term for different forms of calciferol □

2 The active form of vitamin D is 1,25-dihydroxyvitamin D_3 □

3 1,25-dihydroxyvitamin D_3 is also called calcitriol □

4 7-dehydrocholesterol conversion to vitamin D_3 is blocked by sunlight □

5 Cholecalciferol is converted to 25-hydroxycholecalciferol in the liver □

6 25-hydroxycholecalciferol is converted to active vitamin D in the kidney, stimulated by parathyroid hormone (PTH) □

7 Some food sources of vitamin D include milk, eggs, fish liver oils □

8 Calcitonin is the major regulator of vitamin D production in the kidney □

9 Vitamin D acts through an intracellular cytoplasmic receptor □

10 The receptor–Vitamin D complex alters nuclear gene expression □

A Physiological actions of vitamin D include:
- Inhibition of calcium absorption from the GIT □
- Stimulation of calcium resorption from bone □
- Stimulation of proteins mediating Ca^{2+} transport across gut membranes □
- It may promote Ca^{2+} reabsorption in the kidneys □

B Causes of vitamin D deficiency include:
- Ageing □
- Dietary deficiencies □
- Chronic diseases e.g. cancer, diabetes, kidney damage □
- Liver cirrhosis □
- Mutations of the vitamin D receptor □
- Rheumatoid arthritis □
- Scanty clothing □

29 Osteoporosis and Paget's disease of bone

Learning objectives

- Be ready to define osteoporosis
- Know the distinction between primary and secondary osteoporosis
- Be aware of some of the risk factors for osteoporosis, especially those associated with the menopause
- Be able to give an account of the aetiology of osteoporosis
- Be able to list drugs used to treat osteoporosis
- Know what is meant by Paget's disease of bone
- Be able to give an account of symptoms, complications and risk factors for the disease
- Be aware of how it is diagnosed and be able to list the treatments

Mini-glossary

- *Osteoblast*: cell that produces and lays down bone
- *Osteoclast*: cell that resorbs bone
- *Osteoporosis*: loss of bone, resulting in brittle, fragile bone

Definitions of osteoporosis

- Bone disease when bone mineral density (BMD) is clinically reduced with disruption of bone micro-architecture
- Fractures caused by stresses not normally considered capable of causing a fracture
- World Health Organization (WHO) definition (essentials of): bone mineral density 2.5 standard deviations below peak bone mass, using a

20 year old of either sex as the standard, or fractures diagnosed as bone fragility fractures

Classification of osteoporosis

- *Primary osteoporosis* caused by age, e.g. postmenopausal osteoporosis or osteoporosis associated with senility
- *Secondary osteoporosis* caused by other disorders, e.g. rheumatoid arthritis, poor nutrition or GIT malabsorption problems

Occurrence of osteoporosis and risk factors (not comprehensive)

- Alcoholism
- Asian or European ethnic groups
- Bilateral removal of ovaries (oophorectomy)
- Chronically low vitamin D and calcium intake
- Drugs, e.g. prolonged use of glucocorticoids
- Early menopause
- Endocrine problems, e.g. Cushing's syndrome, diabetes, thyrotoxicosis
- Family history of fractures
- Insufficient or excess prolonged physical demand, e.g. sedentary professions and professional athletes respectively
- Low body weight
- Low peak bone mass
- Postmenopausal women, in whom estrogens are low (*see* also below), but also occurs in older men
- Premature ovarian failure
- Prolonged premenstrual amenorrhoea

Diagnosis of osteoporosis

- Dual energy X-ray absorptiometry (DEXA scan)
- Fracture caused by falling from a standing position, regardless of age

Aetiology of osteoporosis

- Healthy bone has a balanced dynamic equilibrium between the activity of osteoblasts laying down bone, and osteoclasts resorbing bone
- Excessive osteoclast activity caused by e.g. age, excessive PTH or glucocorticoids
- Reduced osteoblast activity caused by e.g. deficiency of calcium, estrogen or testosterone, which normally promote osteoblast activity
- The result of excessive osteoclast activity is bone remodelling, which

means abnormal growth patterns in bone, and increased bone porosity, which weakens bone
- Repeated fractures and the process of bone healing also contribute to bone fragility
- The most affected bones are in the wrists, hip (which are serious for older patients), the proximal femur and the spine, and spinal vertebrae, which may cause curvature of the spine

Treatment of osteoporosis

- Preventive with calcium and vitamin D supplements and hormone replacement therapy in women, using synthetic estrogens or selective estrogen receptor modulators (SERMs), e.g. raloxifene
- Bisphosphonates, e.g. sodium alendronate or risendronate, which reduce the rate of bone turnover, partly by slowing down bone resorption
- Teriparatide, a recombinant fraction of PTH, is used mainly in patients who cannot take bisphosphonates or who have already suffered fractures
- Calcitonin is sometimes prescribed as part of treatment for osteoporosis
- Oral strontium ranelate, an example of a newer class of drug called a dual action bone agent (DUBA), which stimulates osteoblast activity while inhibiting osteoclast activity

Paget's disease of bone[1]

What is it?

- A disorder of bone remodelling when the equilibrium between osteoclast and osteoblast activity becomes disturbed and new bone is laid down and existing bone resorbed without reference to the requirements of normal bone maintenance

What are the symptoms and complications of the disease?

- Bone and joint pain, often due to nerve compression caused by growing bone
- Swelling and inflammation (reddening) at joints
- Bowing of the upper leg
- Abnormal skull shape
- Fractures, especially of the femur, pelvis, skull, spine and tibia
- Sometimes the patient remains symptom-free until routine X-rays reveal the presence of the disease
- Greater incidence of heart problems due to high metabolic demands
- Arthritis can result
- Low risk of bone cancer (<1%) of patients

---

[1] Not to be confused with Paget's disease of the nipple.

Who is most at risk?

- Both sexes are equally at risk.
- Paget's disease of bone usually affects those in their 50s or older.

How is it diagnosed?

- X-ray, which shows up abnormal bone shape due to abnormally high or low bone deposition
- Bone scans using radioactive isotopes, e.g. gallium-67, which becomes concentrated in bone affected by Paget's disease, and which is visualised in bone as a darker area
- Raised blood levels of alkaline phosphatase, a marker of bone turnover

How is Paget's disease of bone treated?

- No treatment may be given if the patient is unaffected
- Treatment for pain if necessary
- Bisphosphonates
- Calcitonin, but largely displaced by bisphosphonates
- Surgery in the case of deformity or joint damage

Chapter 29 quiz

Answer T (true) or F (false)

1 An osteoblast is a cell that resorbs bone

2 Osteoporosis is the loss of bone causing fragile, brittle bones

3 Primary osteoporosis is considered to be caused by ageing

4 Secondary osteoporosis is caused by other health problems

5 Diagnosis of osteoporosis uses DEXA scans and through fractures from falls when standing

6 Paget's disease is a disorder of bone remodelling

7 Paget's disease occurs predominantly in women

A Treatment of osteoporosis is mainly:
- Preventive with calcium and vitamin D supplements
- HRT using synthetic estrogens or SERMs
- Use of bisphosphonates, e.g. sodium alendronate
- Teriparatide, an analogue of PTH
- Calcitonin as a supplement to other treatments
- Oral strontium ranelate

B Symptoms of osteoporosis may include:
- Loss of sensation in bone and joints
- Inflammation and swelling at joints
- Abnormal skull shape
- Heart problems
- Fractures

C Paget's disease is diagnosed using:
- X-ray
- Bone scans using radioactive isotopes e.g. gallium-67
- Blood levels of alkaline phosphatase, which is reduced in Paget's disease

D Paget's disease may be treated:
- With nothing if the patient is unaffected
- For pain if needed
- With bisphosphonates
- Surgically if there is bone damage or deformity

30 Multiple endocrine neoplasia

Learning objectives
Mini-glossary
Definition of multiple endocrine neoplasia (MEN)
MEN type 1
MEN type 2
Treatment and prognosis for multiple endocrine neoplasia

Learning objectives

- Know the definition of MEN
- Be able to distinguish the differences given between the different forms of MEN

Mini-glossary

- *Autosomal dominant disorder:* a disorder when affected patients have, on a pair of autosomal chromosomes, one copy of a normal gene from one parent and one copy of the mutant gene from the other parent, where the mutant gene is dominant
- *Autosomal recessive disorder:* a genetic, inherited disease or condition that occurs only in patients who have received two copies of an autosomal mutant gene, one from each parent, where the mutant gene is recessive
- *Autosome:* any chromosome other than a sex chromosome
- *Neuroma:* tumour derived from a nerve cell

Definition of multiple endocrine neoplasia (MEN)

- Also termed multiple endocrine adenomatosis (MEA)
- The term 'multiple endocrine neoplasia' covers three endocrine syndromes, inherited as autosomal dominant disorders, when there are co-existing tumours of endocrine glands, each of which has its own characteristic features

MEN type 1

- Also called Wermer's syndrome
- Glands affected:
  - *parathyroid:* parathyroid tumour, resulting in hyperparathyroidism

- *pancreas:* pancreatic islet cell tumour, resulting in hyperinsulinaemia, gastrinoma (Zollinger–Ellison syndrome) and hypoglycaemia
- *pituitary:* pituitary adenoma, which may result in over-secretion of any of the pituitary hormones

MEN type 2

- Also called Sipple syndrome and subdivided into 2A and 2B

MEN type 2A

- Glands affected:
  - *thyroid:* medullary thyroid cancer, causing over-secretion of calcitonin
  - *adrenal:* phaeochromocytoma, which is a tumour secreting catechol-amines
  - *parathyroid:* parathyroid tumours, secreting PTH

MEN type 2A

- Glands affected (similar to 2A with added features):
  - *adrenal:* phaeochromocytoma, which is a tumour secreting catechol-amines
  - *thyroid:* medullary thyroid cancer, causing over-secretion of calcitonin
- Mucosal neuromas (tumours, usually in the upper GIT, and sometimes on the oral mucosa)
- Marfanoid features: symptoms of Marfan's syndrome, which is a disease of connective tissue resulting in, e.g. tallness, long, thin fingers and toes, heart problems and partial dislocation of the lenses of the eyes

Treatment and prognosis for multiple endocrine neoplasia

- There is no cure for this genetic disease.
- Surgery maybe used to remove a phaeochromocytoma.
- Some authorities believe there may be a case in some patients for thyroidectomy and replacement with thyroid hormone.
- The prognosis is complicated by the occurrence of cancer metastases, and radiotherapy and chemotherapy may not halt the spread of the cancer.
- MEN 2B is the most dangerous form.
- Early diagnosis increases the survival potential.
- Some patients with MEN 2A will not exhibit any symptoms at all, and the availability of a screening tool for early diagnosis may improve survival rates.

Chapter 30 quiz

Answer T (true) or F (false)

1　An autosome is a sex chromosome ☐

2　A neuroma is a tumour derived from a nerve cell ☐

3　MEN type 1 is also called Werner's syndrome ☐

4　MEN type 1 affects the thyroid, pancreas and pituitary ☐

5　MEN type 2 is also called the Sipple syndrome ☐

6　MEN type 2 is further subdivided into 2A and 2B ☐

7　MEN 2B is the most dangerous ☐

A　MEN 2A includes:

- Medullary thyroid cancer ☐
- Phaeochromocytoma ☐
- Parathyroid tumours, secreting calcitonin ☐

B　MEN 2B includes:

- Phaeochromocytoma ☐
- Medullary thyroid cancer ☐
- Mucosal neuromas ☐
- Marfanoid features[1] ☐

[1] Marfan's syndrome: a disease of connective tissue.

Answers to the quizzes

Chapter 2

1 Endocrine hormones are produced by ductless glands ☐T☐

2 Paracrine hormones act on cells that produce them ☐T☐

3 The pituitary gland is situated below the sella turcica ☐F☐

   It is found *in* the sella turcica

4 ACTH releases adrenal medullary hormones ☐F☐

   It releases *adrenocortical hormones*

5 Corticotrophin releases ACTH ☐F☐

   Corticotrophin *is* ACTH

6 FSH promotes LH secretion ☐F☐

7 The thyroid gland is located in front of the trachea ☐T☐

8 Calcitonin promotes calcium resorption from bone ☐F☐

   Calcitonin *inhibits* calcium resorption

9 Insulin promotes glucose removal from the blood ☐T☐

10 CCK releases insulin from the pancreas ☐F☐

   CCK releases *glucagon* from the pancreas

11 Ghrelin promotes feeding behaviour ☐T☐

12 Motilin contracts upper gut muscles ☐T☐

13 Erythropoietin promotes red blood cell production ☐T☐

14 Relaxin is produced by the ovary ☐T☐

15 High HDL is a risk factor for atherosclerosis ☐F☐

   High *LDL* is a risk factor

16 The term iatrogenic describes treatment-induced disease ☐T☐

17 Vitamin D is not produced by the kidney ☐F☐

   It *is* produced by the kidney

18 Craniopharyngiomas are brain tumours ☐T☐

19 Prolactinomas can be treated with a dopamine antagonist ☐F☐

   They are treated with a dopamine *agonist*

20 Thyrotoxicosis is caused by excessive thyroid secretion ☐T☐

21 Laron's dwarfism is the result of a GH receptor defect ☐T☐

22 Cushing's syndrome is due to excessive androgen production ☐F☐

   It is due to excessive *glucocorticoid* production

23 Phaeochromocytoma is a catecholamine-secreting tumour ☐T☐

24 Endocrine hypertension may result from low DOC production ☐F☐

   It may result from *high* DOC production

25 Obesity is associated with type II diabetes ☐T

26 Digoxin toxicity is enhanced by calcium ☐T

27 Osteomalacia is excessive bone mineralisation ☐F
It is *defective* bone matrix mineralisation

28 Chronic GnRH treatment promotes gonadotrophin secretion ☐F
Chronic GnRH treatment *inhibits* gonadotrophin secretion

29 Precocious puberty may be treated with progestational steroids ☐T

30 Insulin-dependent diabetes is treated with oral hypoglycaemic drugs ☐F
IDDM is treated with *insulin*

A Insulin:
- Is released from islet cells in the pancreas ☐T
- Inhibits glucose uptake into cells ☐F
Insulin *promotes* glucose uptake into cells
- Release is enhanced by gastric inhibitory peptide ☐T
- Release is impaired in obesity ☐T
- Is used in insulin-independent diabetes mellitus ☐T
- Is taken orally in tablet form ☐F
Oral insulin tablets are still being developed

B The anterior pituitary gland:
- Secretes oxytocin and vasopressin ☐T
- Secretes ACTH under the control of CRH ☐T
- Controls thyroid function by secreting TRH ☐F
It controls thyroid function by secreting *TSH*
- Secretion of LH is inhibited by progesterone ☐T

C The hypothalamus:
- Secretes somatostatin ☐T
- Synthesises oxytocin and vasopressin ☐T
- Can develop tumours affecting growth ☐T
- Controls anterior pituitary endocrine function through nervous connections ☐F
It controls pituitary endocrine function through the *portal blood system*

D The anterior pituitary gland secretes:
- ACTH ☐T
- Somatostatin ☐T
- Ghrelin ☐F
Ghrelin is secreted by the *GIT*
- Dopamine ☐F
Dopamine is released from the *brain* and inhibits pituitary prolactin release

E   Hypothalamic–pituitary dysfunction in adults is usually due to:

- Craniopharyngiomas   F
  This is more usual in *children*
- Infarction of pituitary blood vessels   T
- Hypersecreting pituitary adenomas   T

F   Hyperprolactinaemia:

- Can be treated with a dopamine agonist   T
- Is under-secretion of prolactin   F
  It is *over-secretion* of prolactin
- Is a possible indicator of a pituitary problem   T

G   Endocrine-related short stature:

- May be due to prolonged treatment with glucocorticoids   T
- Is a result of precocious puberty   T
- May be caused by a GH mutation   F
  It may be caused by a GH *receptor* mutation
- Is treated with GH until epiphyseal closure   T

H   Endocrine hypertension may result from:

- Phaeochromocytoma   T
- Deficient DOC production   F
- Abnormally high aldosterone secretion   F
- Cushing's syndrome   T
- Primary aldosteronism   T

Chapter 3

1   Cyclic AMP is a second messenger for epinephrine   T
2   Aminophylline causes bronchiolar constriction   F
   Aminophylline dilates bronchioles
3   Amenorrhoea can be caused by 11β-hydroxylase deficiency   T
4   Diffusion requires energy   F
   Diffusion requires only a concentration gradient
5   Active transport utilises ATP for energy   T
6   Glucose is transported into the cell by facilitated transport   T
7   Neurosecretion is a property of pituitary cells   F
   Neurosecretion is a property of neurones which secrete chemicals
8   Paracrine cells secrete hormones acting on neighbouring cells   T
9   GnRH is a neuroendocrine hormone   T
10 Estradiol works mainly through intracellular receptors   T

11 Dopamine stimulates prolactin release from the anterior pituitary — F
Dopamine *inhibits* prolactin release

12 Acetylcholinesterase inactivates ACh in the presynaptic nerve terminal — F
Acetylcholinesterase inactivates ACh in the postsynaptic nerve terminal

13 Presynaptic autoreceptors usually inhibit further release of a
neurotransmitter — T

14 Diltiazem is a potassium channel blocker — F
Diltiazem is a *calcium* channel blocker

Chapter 4

A   Biofeedback:
- Is a form of nourishment — F
- Is a biosysytem controlling a set point, e.g. hormone levels — T

B   A negative feedback system:
- Increases the value of the set point — F
- Decreases the value of the set point — T

C   Biofeedback mechanisms control:
- Fertility — T
- Metabolism — T
- Human sexual behaviour — F
Humans have voluntary control
- Adrenal hormones — T
- Salt and water balance — T

D   The components of a biofeedback system include:
- A signal — T
- A transducer — T
- A sensor — T
- A responder — T

E   *See* p. 32
F   *See* p. 32
G   *See* p. 33

Chapter 5

1 GHRH releases GH from the posterior pituitary — F
GHRH releases GH from the anterior pituitary

2 GH stimulates gluconeogenesis in muscle — T

3 GH directly stimulates bone growth — F
GH indirectly stimulates bone growth through IGF-1

4 The growth hormone receptor activates intracellular kinases ⬚T

5 GH release is inhibited by pituitary somatostatin ⬚F

   GH release is inhibited by hypothalamic somatostatin

6 GH deficiency in children causes failure to grow ⬚T

7 GH deficiency is usually caused by hypothalamic–pituitary malfunction ⬚T

8 In children treatment is with GH until adulthood ⬚F

   Treatment is stopped when growth is complete

9 GH excess is usually caused by bacterial infection ⬚F

   GH excess is usually caused by pituitary adenoma

10 GH excess causes gigantism in children ⬚T

11 Acromegaly results from excess GH in adults ⬚T

12 Acromegaly results in diabetes in all patients ⬚F

   In _some_ patients diabetes occurs through lowered glucose tolerance

13 Acromegaly results in enlargement of the upper mandible ⬚F

   Acromegaly results in enlargement of the _lower_ mandible

14 GH excess is treated with dopamine agonists and surgery or radiation to remove tumours ⬚T

Chapter 6

A   Normal growth and final height attainment depend on:

- Normally functioning gonads in early childhood ⬚F

   They depend on normally functioning gonads during the pubertal growth spurt

- Adequate secretion of growth hormone ⬚T
- Normal thyroid function in the early postnatal period ⬚T
- Adequate secretion of IGF-1 during the period of growth ⬚T
- Genetic factors ⬚T

B   Impaired growth may be due to:

- Insufficient intellectual stimulation during early childhood ⬚F

   There is no convincing evidence for this yet

- Chronic diseases which impair food absorption ⬚T
- Prolonged treatment with glucocorticoids during childhood ⬚T
- Poor nutrition during growth ⬚T
- Thyroid over-activity during growth ⬚F

   It may be due to thyroid _under-activity_ during growth

C   Symptoms and features of growth failure include:

- Hirsutism ⬚F

   Hirsutism is a symptom of androgen activity

- Growth velocity less than 6 cm per year ⬚T

- Reduced muscle mass   `T`
- Skeletal abnormalities caused by GH deficiency   `T`
- High-pitched voice   `T`
- Height less than the second percentile   `F`
  Height less than the *third* percentile is a feature

D   Treatment of impaired growth involves:

- Diagnosis of cause   `T`
- Treatment with recombinant sex hormones   `F`
- Treatment with recombinant GH   `T`
- Regular comparison with standard growth curves   `T`
- Treatment until epiphyseal closure   `T`

E   Monitoring during treatment involves:

- Regular IQ tests   `F`
- Measurement of serum IGF-1 and IGFBP-3   `T`
- Measurement of plasma haemoglobin   `F`
- Measurement of serum bone alkaline phosphatase   `T`
- Regular assessment of bone age advancement   `T`

Chapter 7

1   Androgens are hormones responsible for the male attributes   `T`
2   Estrogens are hormones responsible for female attributes   `T`
3   Progesterone is not necessary for implantation   `F`
    Progesterone *is* necessary for implantation
4   Corticosteroids are synthesised in the adrenal medulla   `F`
    Steroids are synthesised in the adrenal cortex
5   Aldosterone is synthesised mainly in the zona fasciculata   `F`
    Aldosterone is synthesised mainly in the zona glomerulosa
6   HCG stimulates progesterone production by the feto-placental unit   `T`
7   17α-hydroxylase converts pregnenolone to 17α-hydroxypregnenolone   `T`
8   11β-hydroxylase converts 17α-hydroxyprogesterone to cortisol   `F`
    11β-hydroxylase converts 11-deoxycortisol to cortisol
9   Testosterone can be converted to estradiol   `T`
10 Cortisol is converted directly to aldosterone in the zona glomerulosa   `F`
    Corticosterone is converted to aldosterone in the zona glomerulosa
11 Over-stimulation by ACTH causes adrenocortical hyperplasia   `T`
12 Steroidogenic enzyme deficiencies can result in failure of puberty `T`
13 Over-stimulation by ACTH can result in hypertension   `T`
14 11β-hydroxylase deficiency can result in virilisation   `T`

15 StAR deficiency is the commonest steroidogenic enzyme deficiency ☐F

StAR deficiency is the *rarest* steroidogenic enzyme deficiency

Chapter 8

A Genetic sex:
- Is determined by the sex chromosomes ☐T
- Determines the secondary sexual characteristics ☐F
- Defines the genotype ☐T

B The phenotype refers to:
- The genetic constitution of the individual ☐F
- The observable secondary sexual characteristics ☐T

C The Sry antigen:
- Is on the X chromosome ☐F
- Switches on genes responsible for testis development ☐T

D Secondary sexual characteristics include:
- The ovary ☐F
- Muscular configuration ☐T
- Hair distribution ☐T
- Accessory sex organs ☐T
- External genitalia ☐T

E In the absence of a testis:
- The male phenotype still develops ☐F
- The female internal secondary sex organs develop ☐T

F The female Müllerian ducts give rise to:
- The ovary ☐F
- The Wolffian ducts ☐F

The Wolffian ducts develop into male accessory sex organs
- The fallopian tubes, uterus and part of the vagina ☐T

G In the presence of a testis:
- The Müllerian ducts atrophy ☐T
- The Wolffian ducts atrophy ☐F
- Testosterone is produced ☐T
- The ductus deferens, epididymis and seminal vesicles develop ☐T

H In the absence of both ovary and testis:
- The Wolffian ducts develop ☐F

The Wolffian ducts *atrophy*
- The Müllerian ducts continue to develop ☐T

I   Klinefelter's syndrome:

- Occurs when males have an extra Y chromosome ☐ F

  Males have an extra X chromosome

- Is characterised by infertility and gynaecomastia ☐ T

- Is characterised by enlarged testis and penis ☐ F

  Testis and penis size are *reduced*

- Causes reduced testosterone and sperm production ☐ T

J   Turner's syndrome:

- Is a genetic defect when women possess an extra X chromosome ☐ F

  Women possess only one X chromosome

- Results in:

  – absence of external genitalia ☐ F

  External genitalia are present

  – absence of ovaries ☐ T

  – webbing of the neck ☐ T

  – short stature ☐ T

  – infertility ☐ T

K   Individuals with true hermaphroditism:

- Possess both ovarian and testicular tissue ☐ T

- Feature breast development and virilisation ☐ T

- May be treated by sex assignment, depending on chromosomal karyotype ☐ T

L   Congenital adrenal hyperplasia:

- Is the most common cause of ambiguous external genitalia ☐ T

- Occurs due to the absence of the testis ☐ F

  Congenital adrenal hyperplasia occurs due to mutations in one or more steroidogenic enzymes

Chapter 9

1   Adrenarche is cessation of adrenal androgen production in girls ☐ F

   Adrenarche is the onset of adrenal androgen production in girls

2   True precocious puberty is caused by inappropriate gonadotrophin release from the pituitary gland ☐ T

3   Pseudoprecocious puberty is caused by ectopic secretion of sex hormones or gonadotrophins ☐ T

A   Male puberty is characterised by:

- Enlargement of the larynx and vocal cord thickening ☐ T

- Penis and scrotum pigmentation ☐ T

- Growth of accessory sex organs ☐ T

- Rise in plasma HDL   `F`
  There is a *fall* in plasma HDL
- Acceleration of linear growth   `T`
- Onset of spermatogenesis   `T`
- Increased androgen activity   `T`

B Female puberty is characterised by:
- Increased CNS sensitivity to negative feedback by estrogen   `F`
  There is *decreased* sensitivity of the CNS to negative feedback by estrogen
- Increased pituitary sensitivity to hypothalamic GnRH   `T`
- Increased production and secretion of estrogen by the ovarian corpus luteum   `F`
  Not the ovarian corpus luteum, but the ovarian *follicle*
- Breast development and a female pattern of fat deposition   `T`

C Sexual infantilism may be due to:
- Anorexia nervosa   `T`
- Congenital overproduction of GnRH   `F`
  It is due to a congenital *deficiency* of GnRH (Kallman's syndrome)
- CNS or pituitary tumours   `T`
- Childhood obesity   `T`
- Other endocrine problems e.g. Cushing's disease   `T`
- Drug treatments e.g. use of cytotoxic drugs   `T`

D Treatment of sexual infantilism and delayed puberty involves:
- Identification of a possible lesion, e.g. tumour   `T`
- Hormonal replacement to mimic the normal situation   `T`
- Follow-up monitoring of pubertal changes and more treatment if necessary   `T`
- Permanent hormonal regime establishment if needed   `T`

E Hormonal therapy for girls may involve:
- Treatment with a GnRH antagonist   `F`
  It involves treatment with pulsatile GnRH
- Treatment with synthetic oral estrogens to induce 'breakthrough' bleeding   `T`
- Establishment of estrogen–progestogen regimes to mimic cyclic hormonal release   `T`

F Hormonal therapy for boys may involve:
- Treatment with implants of GnRH   `F`
  GnRH implants actually produce sterility; GnRH should be *pulsatile*
- Long-acting testosterone analogues   `T`

Chapter 10

1 The ovarian functions are mainly sex hormone and ovum production   T
2 Follicles develop in the cortex of the ovary   T
3 The fertilised egg is implanted in the uterine myometrium   F
4 The fimbria conduct eggs to the uterus   F
5 Menses occurs just before menstrual flow   F
6 The mature follicle is called a Graafian follicle   T
7 FSH promotes conversion of androgens to estrogens in the ovary   T
8 FSH inhibits follicular growth   F
9 The follicular (proliferative) phase lasts about 8–11 days   T
10 Ovulation lasts about 1 hour   F
11 The luteal (secretory) phase lasts about 13–15 days   T
12 Estradiol stimulates progesterone receptor synthesis   T
13 Estrogen stimulates inhibin secretion in the ovarian granulosa cell   T
14 Inhibin inhibits pituitary secretion of FSH   T
15 Amenorrhoea is abnormally frequent menstrual periods   F
16 Dysmenorrhoea is painful menstruation   T
17 Secondary dysmenorrhoea affects mainly younger women   F
18 Menorrhagia is abnormally heavy bleeding during menstruation   T
19 Metrorrhagia is unexpected bleeding from the vagina outside normally expected periods and should always be investigated   T

Chapter 11

1 Estradiol causes epiphyseal closure at puberty   T
2 Estradiol is responsible for the female pattern of fat distribution   T
3 Estradiol inhibits progesterone receptor synthesis   F
   Estradiol *promotes* progesterone receptor synthesis
4 In pregnancy, estradiol limits bodily fluid retention   F
   In pregnancy estradiol *promotes* fluid retention
5 Estradiol increases plasma LDL   F
6 Estradiol enhances fluid retention   T
7 Estradiol stimulates myometrial oxytocin receptor synthesis   T
8 Estradiol promotes calcium resorption from bone   F
   Estradiol *inhibits* calcium resorption from bone
9 Estradiol decreases bowel motility   T
10 SERMs are selective estrogen receptor agonists   F
   SERMS are selective estrogen receptor *modulators*
11 Aromatase inhibitors block conversion of androgens to estrogens   T
12 Estrogens are known to worsen breast cancer   T

13 SERMs and aromatase inhibitors are indicated for estrogen receptor-
   positive biopsies   T

14 Estrogen loss may be implicated in postmenopausal osteoporosis   T

15 Estrone is a powerful estrogen   F
   Estrone is a *weak* estrogen

A Progesterone:
   • Is essential for pregnancy to be maintained   T
   • Is produced by the ovarian follicle before ovulation   F
     Progesterone is produced by the ovarian corpus luteum *after* ovulation
   • Enhances cellular sensitivity to insulin   T
   • Produces a secretory post-ovulatory uterine endothelium   T
   • Promotes alveolobular development in the breast   T
   • Decreases body temperature   F
     Progesterone increases body temperature

B Refer to Figure 11.1, p. 74, for the correct labelling of this figure

Chapter 12

A Important functions of progesterone in pregnancy are:
   • It prepares the endometrium for blastocyst implantation   T
   • It is necessary for formation of the cervical mucus plug   T
   • Stimulation of endometrial secretions   T
   • It enhances the contractility of endometrial muscle   F
     Progesterone *inhibits* contractility of endometrial muscle
   • It has an important role in preparing mammary glands for lactation T

B Estriol:
   • Maternal plasma levels normally fall as pregnancy progresses   F
     Maternal levels progressively *rise* during pregnancy
   • Is synthesised by the fetal adrenal gland   T
   • Secretion by the fetus is controlled by fetal TRH   F
     Secretion is not controlled by fetal TRH but by fetal *ACTH*
   • Levels therefore reflect the health of the fetal pituitary   T

C Human chorionic gonadotrophin (HCG):
   • Is structurally related to FSH   F
     HCG is not related to FSH but to *LH*
   • Is an indicator of pregnancy   T
   • Is detected in the second trimester   F
     **It is detected 8–10 days after fertilisation – hence it is diagnostic for
     pregnancy**
   • Is synthesised by the syncytiotrophoblast   T

- Prevents destruction of the corpus luteum $\boxed{\text{T}}$
- Stimulates luteal progesterone production $\boxed{\text{T}}$
- Stimulates testosterone production by the fetus $\boxed{\text{T}}$

D Human placental lactogen (HPL):
- Is structurally similar to growth hormone and prolactin $\boxed{\text{T}}$
- Is synthesised by the corpus luteum $\boxed{\text{F}}$
  It is synthesised by the syncytiotrophoblast
- Is initially detected 2–5 weeks after fertilisation in fetal blood $\boxed{\text{F}}$
  It is detected in maternal but *not* fetal blood
- Reported effects include:
  - diabetogenic $\boxed{\text{T}}$
  - contributes to insulin resistance of pregnancy $\boxed{\text{T}}$
  - increased availability of amino acids and glucose $\boxed{\text{T}}$

E Relaxin:
- Is structurally similar to insulin $\boxed{\text{T}}$
- Is synthesised mainly in the decidual lining of the uterus $\boxed{\text{F}}$
  It is synthesised *mainly* in the corpus luteum and placenta
- Is initially detected when HCG levels start to rise $\boxed{\text{T}}$
- Synergises with progesterone to inhibit uterine motility $\boxed{\text{T}}$
- Relaxes connective tissue of the pubic symphysis at birth $\boxed{\text{T}}$

F Parturition:
- Is the onset and course of labour and birth $\boxed{\text{T}}$
- In humans is initiated by a rise in fetal cortisol $\boxed{\text{F}}$
  In *sheep* parturition is initiated by a rise in fetal cortisol; the cause of initiation in humans is unknown at the time of writing
- Is associated with increased oxytocin production by the fetus $\boxed{\text{T}}$
- Is facilitated by increased uterine contractility $\boxed{\text{T}}$
- Is accompanied by a sharp fall in plasma progesterone $\boxed{\text{T}}$
- Is accompanied by a sharp rise in nitric oxide synthase activity $\boxed{\text{T}}$

G Prolactin:
- Is synthesised by lactotroph cells in the posterior pituitary $\boxed{\text{F}}$
  It is synthesised in lactotroph cells in the *anterior* pituitary
- Release is stimulated by dopamine $\boxed{\text{F}}$
  Release is *inhibited* by dopamine (prolactin-inhibitory factor (PIF))
- Stimulates milk production in the breast $\boxed{\text{T}}$
- Suppresses fertility during suckling $\boxed{\text{T}}$
- Levels are raised in stress $\boxed{\text{T}}$
- Suppresses testosterone synthesis and spermatogenesis $\boxed{\text{T}}$

Chapter 13

1 Monophasic oral contraceptives have a variable estrogen dose ☐F

   Monophasic OCs have fixed estrogen dose

2 Monophasic oral contraceptives have fixed doses of estrogen + progestogen ☐T

3 Estrogen's contraceptive action is through blocking LH release ☐F

   Estrogen blocks FSH release, thus inhibiting follicle development

4 Progestogens inhibit preovulatory LH release ☐T

5 Progestogen changes cervical mucus consistency ☐T

6 The COCP efficacy is estimated to be 95% ☐F

   It is 99.9%

7 Higher doses of estrogen are associated with an increased risk of venous thromboembolism ☐T

8 COCPs may reduce the risks of colonic, endometrial and epithelial cancers ☐T

9 COCP efficacy may be reduced by drugs which induce liver microsomal enzymes, e.g. rifampicin ☐T

10 Low-dose COCPs do not reduce the risk of breast cancer ☐F

   Low-dose OCs may be associated with a lower risk of breast cancer

11 Combined OCs used for more than 5 years may increase cervical cancer risk ☐T

12 There is no risk of liver cancer with long-term use ☐F

   There is *increased* risk of liver cancer with long-term use

13 There is increased risk of breast cancer with COCPs ☐T

A Adverse effects of COCPs (especially within the first 3 months) include:

- Weight gain ☐T
- Breakthrough bleeding ☐T
- Diarrhoea, nausea and vomiting ☐T
- Headache ☐T
- Dysmenorrhoea ☐F

   The COCP may actually *reduce* the risks of dysmenorrhoea

B Risks associated with the COCP include:

- Myocardial infarction and stroke in older women and smokers ☐T
- Ischaemic stroke and haemorrhage ☐T
- Risks of ischaemic stroke in smokers ☐T
- Venous thromboembolism in women:
  - who smoke ☐T
  - who are older ☐T
  - after surgery ☐T
  - who are obese ☐T
  - with malignancy ☐T

C   The progestogen-only pill:

- Cannot be prescribed for women in whom the combined OC is contraindicated   F

  It *can* be prescribed for these women, depending on individual history

- Should be taken at the same time each day to maximise contraceptive cover   T
- May increase ectopic pregnancy risk if taken at time of fertilisation   T
- May cause appetite and weight changes   T
- May have central effects, e.g. mild sedation, dizziness   T
- Is associated with increased risk of benign ovarian cysts   T
- Is contraindicated:
  - in pregnancy   T
  - in porphyria   T
  - in undiagnosed vaginal bleeding   T
  - in gonadotrophin-secreting tumours   T
  - in liver disorders, e.g. liver adenoma   T
  - if there is no recurrence of breast cancer after 5 years   F

  The POP can be used 5 years after breast cancer if there is no recurrence of cancer

D   Advantages of parenteral progestogen contraception are:

- It avoids the problem of missing a dose   T
- It may alleviate problems, e.g. PMS, dysmenorrhoea   T
- It reduces pelvic infection risks   T
- There is a rapid return to fertility after the injection wears off   F

  Fertility return rate is variable, unpredictable and may be delayed for several months

E   Disadvantages of emergency contraception include:

- Danger of an ectopic pregnancy   T
- A prescription is needed   T
- It is less effective than an IUD   T
- It can cause nausea and vomiting (with loss of drug)   T
- It may change the timing of the next menses   T
- Need for barrier contraception until the following menses   T
- Reduced efficacy if taken with enzyme-inducing drugs   T

F   Advantages of progestogen-only IUDs are:

- They can be used in pregnancy   F

  All IUDS are contraindicated in pregnancy

- A long period of contraceptive cover   T
- Rapid restoration of fertility after removal   T
- Virtually all hormonal effects are local   T

- They reduce the risk of pelvic inflammatory disease   T
- They are an option for women with heavy menses   T
14 *See* p. 93 for answers

Chapter 14

A   Menopause:

- Is interruption of menstruation   F
  Menopause is generally accepted to have occurred if 12 months elapse without menstruation
- Is cessation of menstruation   T
- Always has an onset after 50 years of age   F
  It can (relatively rarely) occur 10 years earlier
- Is accompanied by reduction and eventual failure of sex hormone production   T
- May be caused in part by failure of the ovaries to respond to LH and FSH   T

B   Symptoms of menopause may include:

- Cardiovascular symptoms, e.g. 'hot flushes' and arrhythmias   T
- Calcification of bone   F
  Symptoms include osteoporosis, i.e. increased *loss* of calcium from bone
- Vaginal dryness and atrophy   T
- Hardening of skin due to cornification   F
  Skin loses plasticity and firmness
- Mood swings   T
- Joint pain, fatigue and insomnia   T
- Urinary incontinence and increased urinary infection risk   T
- Weight loss   F
  Weight gain is more usual
- Increased LDL with raised atherosclerosis risk   T

C   Hormone replacement therapy (HRT) includes:

- Treatment for hypercalcaemia   F
  It includes treatment to supplement calcium and slow bone resorption
- Sex hormone replacement   T
- Counselling   T
- Bed rest   F
  Improved diet and *more* exercise are recommended

D   The main HRT treatments are:

- Low-dose estrogen   T
- Low-dose estrogen + a progestogen   T

- Glucocorticoids | F |

  Glucocorticoids have no rational basis for use here
- Combined conjugated estrogens | T |
- Progestogen alone | T |
- Tibolone | T |

E   The main routes of HRT administration are:

- Nasal sprays containing estradiol | T |
- Topical gels containing estradiol | T |
- Vaginal rings containing estradiol | T |
- Oral low-dose anti-estrogens alone or with a progestogen | F |

  An estrogen not an anti-estrogen is used
- Skin patches containing estradiol, the natural estrogen alone, or with a
  synthetic progestogen | T |

F   Who should not take HRT?

- Patients who are pregnant or breast-feeding | T |
- Those with undiagnosed vaginal bleeding | T |
- Patients with liver disease | T |
- Patients with acne | F |
- Patients with active thrombophlebitis | T |
- Patients with untreated endometrial hyperplasia | T |
- Patients with a history of venous thrombosis | T |
- Patients with any current or recent thromboembolic arterial disorders,
  e.g. angina or myocardial infarction | T |
- Patients with Dubin–Johnson or Rotor's syndromes | T |

G   The main risks associated with HRT are:

- Increased risk of endometrial cancer with the combined estrogen–
  progestogen pill | F |

  **Progestogen inclusion with estrogen *lessens* the risk of endometrial
  cancer**
- Venous thromboembolism and stroke | T |
- Increased breast cancer risk within 1–2 years after starting HRT | T |

  However, risk may lessen within 5 years of stopping HRT
- Increased risk of gallstones and liver damage if used for more than 5 years | T |

Chapter 16

1 Androgens exert a positive feedback effect on gonadotrophin release from
   the anterior pituitary gland | F |

   Androgens exert a *negative* feedback effect

2 5α-dihydrotestosterone is a potent androgenic metabolite of testosterone | T |

3 The Leydig cells of the testis produce the spermatozoa $\boxed{\text{F}}$

The seminiferous tubules produce the spermatozoa

4 Testosterone is necessary for maintenance of the accessory sex organs $\boxed{\text{T}}$

5 The vas deferens conducts spermatozoa from the epididymis to the urethra $\boxed{\text{T}}$

6 The Cowper's glands produce part of the seminal fluid $\boxed{\text{T}}$

7 Androgens also are anabolic $\boxed{\text{T}}$

8 Benign prostatic hyperplasia is treated with radiotherapy $\boxed{\text{F}}$

BPH is benign, and usually requires surgery; drugs used include alpha-blockers and androgen receptor blockers

9 Refer to Figure 16.1, p. 111, for the correct labelling of this figure

A The penis:

- Ejects semen through the proximal portion of the urethra $\boxed{\text{F}}$

  Ejection is through the *distal* portion of the urethra

- Becomes erect during sexual excitement through engorgement with blood $\boxed{\text{T}}$

- Needs to be removed in prostate cancer $\boxed{\text{F}}$

  The *testes* need to be removed to remove testosterone

B The testes:

- Need to be external to the body at a lower temperature to ensure the viability of the spermatozoa $\boxed{\text{T}}$

- Contain Leydig cells which respond to pituitary FSH to synthesise testosterone $\boxed{\text{F}}$

  The Leydig cells respond to *LH* to synthesise testosterone

- Contain seminiferous tubules which produce the spermatozoa under the influence of FSH $\boxed{\text{T}}$

C Androgens, e.g. testosterone:

- Are necessary for spermatogenesis $\boxed{\text{T}}$

- Cause the development of the male sex organs $\boxed{\text{T}}$

- Are necessary for maintenance of the sex organs $\boxed{\text{T}}$

- Promote scalp hair growth $\boxed{\text{F}}$

  Androgens promote *beard* growth but promote scalp hair *loss*

- Cause voice deepening $\boxed{\text{T}}$

- Promote muscle wasting $\boxed{\text{F}}$

  Androgens promote skeletal muscle *development*

Chapter 17

A Oxytocin:

- Is a decapeptide $\boxed{\text{F}}$

  Oxytocin is a nonapeptide

- Is synthesised in the hypothalamus $\boxed{\text{T}}$

- Stimulates milk ejection from the breast $\boxed{\text{T}}$
- Relaxes uterine smooth muscle $\boxed{\text{F}}$
  Oxytocin *contracts* uterine smooth muscle
- Is released from the posterior pituitary $\boxed{\text{T}}$
- Promotes maternal behaviour $\boxed{\text{T}}$
- Receptor synthesis in the uterus rises in late gestation under the influence of estrogen $\boxed{\text{T}}$

B   Oxytocin production and release:
- Are stimulated by an increase in plasma progesterone $\boxed{\text{F}}$
  They are stimulated by a *decrease* in plasma progesterone
- Are stimulated by stretching of the cervix and vagina at birth $\boxed{\text{T}}$
- Are stimulated by stress $\boxed{\text{F}}$
  Oxytocin release is *inhibited* by acute stress

C   Vasopressin:
- Is a nonapeptide structurally related to oxytocin $\boxed{\text{T}}$
- Is also called diuretic hormone $\boxed{\text{T}}$
- Is synthesised mainly in magnocellular neurones of hypothalamic nuclei $\boxed{\text{T}}$
- Is transported through neurosecretory neurones to the posterior pituitary as part of a larger protein called neurophysin II $\boxed{\text{T}}$

D   Important actions of vasopressin include:
- Reabsorption of water from the kidney's collecting ducts $\boxed{\text{T}}$
- Vasodilatation $\boxed{\text{F}}$
  Actions include *vasoconstriction*

E   Central actions of vasopressin *may* include:
- Mediation of social and aggressive behaviour $\boxed{\text{T}}$
- Involvement in memory $\boxed{\text{T}}$
- Involvement in central control of blood pressure and temperature $\boxed{\text{T}}$

F   Failure of vasopressin secretion results in:
- Cranial diabetes insipidus $\boxed{\text{T}}$
- Nephrogenic diabetes insipidus $\boxed{\text{T}}$
- Loss of memory $\boxed{\text{F}}$

G   Treatment of diabetes insipidus includes:
- Balancing fluid intake $\boxed{\text{T}}$
- Administration of vasopressin analogues $\boxed{\text{T}}$
- Diuretics for nephrogenic diabetes insipidus $\boxed{\text{T}}$

Chapter 18

1   Renin is secreted by the kidney in response to a rise in blood pressure $\boxed{\text{F}}$
Renin is released in response to a *fall* in blood pressure

2   Renin is released also in response to a rise in blood osmolarity ⬚T

3   Angiotensin is derived from angiotensinogen ⬚T

4   Renin is an enzyme which converts angiotensin I to angiotensin II ⬚T

5   Angiotensin II is a powerful vasodilator in the kidneys ⬚F
    Angiotensin II is a powerful *vasoconstrictor*

6   Angiotensin II stimulates aldosterone release from the adrenal cortex ⬚T

7   Aldosterone inhibits the re-uptake of Na^+ and water in the kidney ⬚F
    Aldosterone *promotes* re-uptake of Na^+ and water in the kidney

8   The RAA system is activated by haemorrhage and hypotension ⬚T

9   Angiotensinogen is converted to angiotensin I in the lungs ⬚F
    Angiotensin I is converted to angiotensin II in the lungs

A   Angiotensin II:

● Is a potent selective constrictor of efferent glomerular arterioles ⬚T

● Stimulates vasopressin release from the pituitary ⬚T

● Promotes Na^+ reabsorption in the proximal tubules ⬚T

● Acts in the kidney through its AT_1 receptor ⬚T

● Action is terminatd by angiotensinase enzymes ⬚T

B   Angiotensin AT_1 receptor blockers:

● Increase blood pressure by constricting arterioles ⬚F
    Reduce **blood pressure by allowing arteriolar** *dilation*

● Reduce aldosterone production ⬚T

● Reduce vasopressin secretion ⬚T

● Are used to treat hypertension and heart failure ⬚T

● Are used to slow nephropathy of diabetes ⬚T

● Include losartan and eprosartan ⬚T

C   ACE inhibitors:

● Block conversion of angiotensinogen to angiotensin I ⬚F
    ACE inhibitors block conversion of angiotensin I to angiotensin II

● Are used to treat hypertension and heart failure ⬚T

● Include captopril and enalapril ⬚T

D   Refer to Figure 18.1, p. 124, for the correct labelling of this figure

E   Refer to p. 124 for a definition

Chapter 19

A   The adrenal gland:

● Is situated below the kidney ⬚F
    The adrenal gland is situated *above* the kidney

● Contains an outer cortex and inner medulla ⬚T

- The outer layer of the cortex is called the zona glomerulosa — T
- The middle layer is called the zona fasciculata — T
- The inner layer is called the zona reticularis — T

B   Of the adrenal steroids:
- Aldosterone is synthesised mainly in the zona reticularis — F
  Aldosterone is synthesised in the zona glomerulosa
- Cortisol is synthesised mainly in the zona fasciculata — T
- Androgens produced include androstenedione and DHEAS — T

C   The adrenal medulla:
- Is a modified sympathetic ganglion — T
- Consists chiefly of catecholamine-secreting chromaffin cells — T
- Releases epinephrine and norethisterone — F
  Epinephrine and *norepinephrine* are released
- Releases catecholamines through cholinergic stimulation — T
- Surrounds the adrenal cortex — F
  The cortex surrounds the medulla

D   Cortisol:
- Is principally a glucocorticoid — T
- Regulates carbohydrate metabolism — T
- Decreases hepatic gluconeogenesis — F
  Cortisol *increases* hepatic gluconeogenesis
- Promotes muscle and fat breakdown — T
- Inhibits catecholamine release from the nerve terminal — F
  Cortisol *permits* catecholamine release from the nerve terminal
- Facilitates catecholamine-mediated mobilisation of fat for energy — T

E   Cortisol synthesis and release from the adrenal gland:
- Are inhibited by ACTH — F
  Cortisol production is *stimulated* by ACTH
- Are under the control of hypothalamic TRH — F
  They are under the control of hypothalamic *CRH*
- Are controlled through a negative feedback action of cortisol — T

F   Side-effects of long-term, high doses of glucocorticoids include:
- Thinning of the skin and hirsutism — T
- Osteoporosis and oedema — T
- Exaggeration of normal body responses to stress — F
  Side-effects include *suppression* of normal responses to stress
- Suppression of the immune system — T
- Gastric ulcers and hirsutism — T

G   Hormonal actions of epinephrine include:
- Dilatation of cutaneous (skin) arterioles through α_1 receptors   ☐ F

   **Hormonal actions of epinephrine include *constriction* of cutaneous
   arterioles through α_1 receptors**
- Increased rate and force of heart contractions through β_1 receptors   ☐ T
- Bronchiolar tree dilatation through β_2 receptors   ☐ T
- Contraction of GIT smooth muscle through α_2 receptors   ☐ F

   **Hormonal actions of epinephrine include *relaxation* of GIT smooth
   muscle through α_2 receptors**
- Contraction of radial muscles of the eye   ☐ T
- Decreased coagulation time   ☐ T
- Increases in blood haemoglobin   ☐ T

H   Metabolic actions of epinephrine include:
- Increased thermogenesis   ☐ T
- Increased lipolysis   ☐ T
- Increased insulin release   ☐ F

   Metabolic actions of epinephrine include *decreased* insulin release
- Increased glucagon release   ☐ T

I   Refer to Figure 19.2, p. 133, for the correct labelling of this figure
J   Refer to Figure 19.5, p. 136, for the correct labelling of this figure

Chapter 20

A   Primary adrenal insufficiency may be the result of damage to the adrenal
   cortex, caused by (e.g.):
- TB infection   ☐ T
- Metastatic carcinoma   ☐ T
- Autoimmune attack   ☐ T
- Fungal infections   ☐ T
- Pituitary damage   ☐ F

   Pituitary damage may cause *secondary* adrenal insufficiency

B   Symptoms of adrenal insufficiency *may* include:
- Weight gain   ☐ F

   They may include weight loss
- Muscle weakness and fatigue   ☐ T
- Hyperpigmentation   ☐ T
- Addisonian crisis if untreated   ☐ T
- Salt craving   ☐ T
- Hyperglycaemia in children   ☐ F

   There may be *hypoglycaemia*

- Amenorrhoea or dysmenorrhoea ☐T
- Mood depression and irritability ☐T

C Diagnosis of adrenal insufficiency includes:
- Measurement of plasma cortisol levels ☐T
- ACTH-induced cortisol release test ☐T
- Insulin-induced hypoglycaemia challenge ☐T
- If secondary adrenal insufficiency is suspected:
  - CT scan of the pituitary ☐T
  - test of pituitary ability to release other hormones, e.g. TSH ☐T

D Adrenal insufficiency is treated:
- With glucocorticoid replacement ☐T
- With mineralocorticoid replacement if needed ☐T
- With salt replacement for secondary adrenal insufficiency ☐F
  Salt replacement is used for *primary* adrenal insufficiency
- In cases of Addisonian crisis:
  - for life-threatening hyperglycaemia ☐T
  - for hypotension and hyperkalaemia ☐T
  - with hydrocortisone, saline and dextrose IV ☐T

E Cushing's disease:
- Reflects under-production of ACTH by the adrenal gland ☐F
  Cushing's disease reflects *over*-production of ACTH by the *pituitary* gland
- Is usually caused by an ACTH-producing adenoma ☐T

F Cushing's syndrome is the *appearance* of the disease caused by:
- Chronic use of glucocorticoids ☐T
- Adrenal hyperplasia ☐T
- ACTH-independent cortisol-producing tumours ☐T
- Increased cortisol production due to severe depression ☐T
- Alcohol insufficiency ☐F
  It can be caused by chronic alcohol *excess*

G Symptoms of Cushing's disease include:
- Hypotension ☐F
  Symptoms include *hypertension*
- Hirsutism ☐T
- Rounding of the face ('moon face') ☐T
- Male impotence ☐T
- Obesity on the trunk of the body ☐T
- Tendency to bruising ☐T

- Abdominal stretch marks ⟦T⟧
- Diabetes mellitus ⟦T⟧
- Oligomenorrhoea or amenorrhoea ⟦T⟧

H Treatment of Cushing's disease and syndrome (depending on diagnosis) is:
- Pituitary radiotherapy ⟦T⟧
- Surgery to remove pituitary adenoma + post-operative hydrocortisone ⟦T⟧
- Adrenalectomy + permanent steroid replacement ⟦T⟧
- Neuromodulators e.g. GABA agonists, 5-HT antagonists ⟦T⟧
- Dopamine antagonists ⟦F⟧
    Dopamine *agonists* are used, e.g. bromocriptine

I Refer to Figure 20.1, p. 144, for the correct labelling of this figure

Chapter 21

1 Insulin is secreted from the islets of Langerhans ⟦T⟧
2 The α-cells secrete insulin ⟦F⟧
    The β-*cells* secrete insulin
3 Insulin consists of two polypeptide chains ⟦T⟧
4 The chains are connected by nucleic acid bridges ⟦F⟧
    The chains are connected by *disulphide* (S–S) bridges
5 Insulin stimulates glucose uptake into tissues from blood ⟦T⟧
6 Insulin stimulates conversion of glucose to glycogen in the liver ⟦T⟧
7 Insulin stimulates conversion of lipid stores to glucose in fat ⟦F⟧
    Insulin stimulates conversion of glucose to lipid stores in fat
8 Insulin inhibits glycogenolysis, i.e. glycogen breakdown to glucose ⟦T⟧
9 Insulin acts in the hypothalamus to suppress appetite ⟦T⟧
10 Insulin release is stimulated by increased plasma glucose ⟦T⟧
11 Glucose inhibits Ca^{2+} uptake by pancreatic islet cells ⟦F⟧
    Glucose *enhances* Ca^{2+} uptake by pancreatic islet cells
12 Insulin release is blocked by raised plasma glucagon ⟦F⟧
    Insulin release is *stimulated* by raised plasma glucagon
13 Insulin release is stimulated by epinephrine ⟦T⟧
14 Some insulin is degraded in the kidney ⟦T⟧
15 Most insulin is removed via the hepatic portal circulation ⟦T⟧
16 Insulin binds to specific intracellular insulin receptors ⟦F⟧
    Insulin binds to *extracellular* membrane-bound insulin receptors
17 Insulin receptors autophosphorylate themselves ⟦T⟧
18 Type 1 diabetes is insulin-dependent diabetes mellitus ⟦T⟧
19 Type 2 diabetes is also called non-insulin-dependent diabetes ⟦T⟧
    The acronyms IDDM and NIDDM are not now favoured by some

20 Type 2 diabetes presents most commonly in childhood F

Type I diabetes presents most commonly in childhood

21 Type 1 diabetes results from autoimmune destruction of islet cells T

22 Treatment of type 1 diabetes mellitus is with insulin T

23 Type 2 (adult-onset) diabetes is associated with obesity, poor diet and a sedentary lifestyle T

This term is less appropriate now due to increased juvenile obesity

A Failed secretion of insulin results in:

- Hyperglycaemia T
- Glucosuria T
- Polydipsia T
- Hyperphagia T
- Reduction in plasma ketone bodies F

There is a potentially fatal *build-up* of plasma ketone bodies

B Known causes of type 2 diabetes include:

- Obesity, poor diet, sedentary lifestyle T
- Decreased insulin receptors T
- Decreased muscle mass T
- Reduced secretion of insulin T

All these factors are probably interdependent

C Treatment aims for type 2 diabetes mellitus include:

- Increased exercise, no smoking, less alcohol T
- Treat hyperlipidaemia T
- Treat any hypertension T
- Raise blood glucose F

Blood glucose should be *lowered*

D Drug treatment for hyperglycaemia employs:

- Sulphonylureas to decrease insulin secretion F

Sulphonylureas are used to *increase* insulin secretion

- Metformin to enhance glucose metabolism T
- Acarbose to reduce post-prandial glucose T
- Thiazolidinediones to reduce tissue resistance to insulin T
- Statins to reduce hyperlipidaemia T
- Beta-blockers and diuretics to treat hypertension T

E Other serious complications of diabetes include:

- Peripheral neuropathies T
- Peripheral nephropathies T

F   Refer to Figure 21.1, p. 149, for the correct labelling of this figure

Chapter 22

1   Glucagon is synthesised in the α-cells of the islets of Langerhans $\boxed{\text{T}}$
2   Glucagon is released when plasma fatty acids and glucose rise $\boxed{\text{F}}$
     Glucagon is released when plasma fatty acids and glucose *fall*
3   Glucagon release is inhibited when plasma energy substrates rise $\boxed{\text{T}}$
4   Insulin inhibits glucagon release $\boxed{\text{T}}$
5   Glucagon is excreted mainly unchanged in the urine $\boxed{\text{F}}$
     Glucagon is metabolised mainly in the liver and kidneys

A   Glucagon's actions include:
•   Promotion of breakdown of glycogen to glucose in the liver $\boxed{\text{T}}$
•   Promotion of hepatic metabolism of amino acids to glucose $\boxed{\text{T}}$
•   Inhibition of hepatic glycogenesis $\boxed{\text{T}}$
•   Stimulation of free fatty acid conversion to ketone bodies $\boxed{\text{T}}$
•   A limited stimulant action on fat lipolysis $\boxed{\text{T}}$

B   Glucagon's cellular actions include:
•   Binding to a specific intracellular receptor $\boxed{\text{F}}$
     The glucagon receptor is on the *cell membrane*
•   Activation of the cyclic AMP second messenger system $\boxed{\text{T}}$
•   Mobilisation of intracellular Ca^{2+} $\boxed{\text{T}}$
•   Downregulation of its own receptor's expression $\boxed{\text{T}}$

C   Glucagon over-production, e.g. by glucagon-secreting tumours:
•   Produces some symptoms similar to those of diabetes $\boxed{\text{T}}$
•   Causes raised plasma glucose $\boxed{\text{T}}$
•   Causes weight loss $\boxed{\text{T}}$
•   Produces a brown skin rash and a bright red tongue $\boxed{\text{T}}$

D   Treatment of a glucagon-secreting tumour is by:
•   Surgical removal of the tumour $\boxed{\text{T}}$
•   Chemotherapy if the tumour is malignant $\boxed{\text{T}}$
•   Reduction of plasma glucagon with octreotide $\boxed{\text{T}}$
•   Treatment of skin rash with IV amino acids and zinc ointment $\boxed{\text{T}}$

Chapter 23

1   Primary hyperthyroidism originates outside the thyroid gland $\boxed{\text{F}}$
     Primary hyperthyroidism originates *inside* **the thyroid gland**
2   Secondary hyperthyroidism originates outside the thyroid gland $\boxed{\text{T}}$

3 Graves' disease is hyperthyroidism caused by excess iodine in water $\boxed{\text{F}}$

It is caused by circulating immunoglobulins which bind TSH receptors on thyroid cells

A The thyroid gland:
- Is situated behind the trachea $\boxed{\text{F}}$

  The thyroid gland is situated *in front of* the trachea
- Consists of two lobes $\boxed{\text{T}}$
- Has functional units called follicles $\boxed{\text{T}}$
- Secretes thyroxine (T_4) and tri-iodothyronine (T_3) $\boxed{\text{T}}$
- Also contains parafollicular calcitonin-secreting cells $\boxed{\text{T}}$
- Also contains parathyroid glands which secrete thyroxine $\boxed{\text{F}}$

  The parathyroid cells secrete *parathyroid hormone* (PTH)

B The thyroid hormones:
- Decrease the metabolic rate $\boxed{\text{F}}$

  The thyroid hormones *regulate* the metabolic rate
- Maintain body temperature through calorigenesis $\boxed{\text{T}}$
- Generate energy through mitochondrial O_2 consumption $\boxed{\text{T}}$
- Generate energy through ATP synthesis $\boxed{\text{T}}$
- Are essential for the proper functioning of growth hormone $\boxed{\text{T}}$
- Are catabolic through:
  - decreasing the rate of insulin metabolism $\boxed{\text{F}}$

  They *increase* the rate of insulin metabolism
  - stimulation of GIT glucose absorption $\boxed{\text{T}}$
  - stimulation of lipolysis $\boxed{\text{T}}$
  - stimulation of liver glycogenolysis $\boxed{\text{T}}$
  - potentiation of epinephrine's stimulation of glycogenolysis $\boxed{\text{T}}$
- Reduce plasma cholesterol $\boxed{\text{T}}$
- Inhibit vitamin A production $\boxed{\text{F}}$

  Thyroid hormones *promote* vitamin A production

C The key steps in thyroid hormone biosynthesis are:
1 Iodide ion uptake pump from blood into thyroid cells $\boxed{\text{T}}$
2 Oxidation of iodide to iodine (I_2) by the peroxidase enzymes $\boxed{\text{T}}$
3 Reaction of I_2 with tyrosine residues on thyroglobulin $\boxed{\text{T}}$
4 Storage of mono-, di- and tri-iodothyronine and thyroxine in colloid $\boxed{\text{T}}$

D TSH controls thyroid hormone release by:
- Inhibiting the uptake of I^- into the thyroid cell $\boxed{\text{F}}$

  TSH *promotes* uptake of I^-
- Promoting amino acid and carbohydrate uptake into thyroid cells $\boxed{\text{T}}$

- Blocking thyroglobulin synthesis $\boxed{\text{F}}$

  TSH *promotes* thyroglobulin synthesis
- Promoting thyroglobulin transfer from colloid for T_3/T_4 release $\boxed{\text{T}}$
- Promoting T_3/T_4 release into the circulation $\boxed{\text{T}}$

E TSH release from the anterior pituitary:
- Is inhibited by hypothalamic TRH $\boxed{\text{F}}$

  TSH release is *stimulated* by hypothalamic TRH
- Is inhibited by T_3 $\boxed{\text{T}}$
- Is increased when plasma levels of thyroid hormones fall $\boxed{\text{T}}$
- Is increased by high levels of glucocorticoids and dopamine agonists $\boxed{\text{F}}$

  TSH release is *inhibited* by high levels of glucocorticoids and dopamine agonists

F Symptoms of hypothyroidism include:
- Goitre $\boxed{\text{T}}$
- Symptoms of lowered metabolism such as:
  - intolerance to cold $\boxed{\text{T}}$
  - easily fatigued $\boxed{\text{T}}$
  - tachycardia (rapid heartbeat) $\boxed{\text{F}}$

    ***Bradycardia* (slowed heartbeat) is a symptom**
  - mental lethargy $\boxed{\text{T}}$
  - hyponatraemia (lowered blood sodium) $\boxed{\text{T}}$
- Brittle nails $\boxed{\text{T}}$
- Dry, coarsened skin $\boxed{\text{T}}$
- Joint and muscle pain $\boxed{\text{T}}$

G Diagnosis of hypothyroidism may include:
- Measurement of low circulating T_3 and T_4 $\boxed{\text{T}}$
- Low circulating TSH $\boxed{\text{F}}$

  Plasma TSH will be *raised* due to loss of negative feedback of T_3
- Raised plasma antibodies to thyroid peroxidase and thyroglobulin $\boxed{\text{T}}$

H Treatment of hypothyroidism involves:
- T_3 or T_4 $\boxed{\text{T}}$
- Dietary iodine supplements if necessary $\boxed{\text{T}}$

I Symptoms of Graves' disease include:
- Exophthalmos (protruding eyeballs) $\boxed{\text{T}}$
- Clubbed fingers $\boxed{\text{T}}$
- Non-pitting oedema $\boxed{\text{T}}$

J The main symptoms of hyperthyroidism may include:
- Raised circulating T_3 and T_4 $\boxed{\text{T}}$

- Hyperthermia and sweating — T
- Exophthalmos — T
- Nervousness and tremor — T
- Easily fatigued — T
- Increased appetite coupled with weight loss — T
- Abnormal sensitivity to cold — F

  There is abnormal sensitivity to *heat*

K Treatment of thyrotoxicosis involves drugs, including:
- Thiourylenes, e.g. carbimazole — T
- Radioactive iodine — T
- Aqueous iodine solution — T
- α_1-blockers — F

  β-*blockers*, e.g. propranolol, are used

Chapter 24

1 Endocrine hypertension has no known cause — F

   It is usually the result of inappropriate endocrine hormone release

2 Endocrine hypertension is often curable — T

3 Either hyperthyroidism or hypothyroidism could cause hypertension — T

4 Diabetes mellitus can cause hypertension — T

5 Over-activity of the RAA system can cause hypertension — T

6 Pregnancy provides protection against hypertension — F

   Pregnancy can *induce* hypertension, perhaps through estrogen effects

A Risks with chronic hypertension include:
- Stroke — T
- Myocardial infarction — T
- Heart failure — T
- Kidney failure — T

B Endocrine disorders often associated with endocrine hypertension include:
- Congenital adrenal hyperplasia — T
- Disorders of glucocorticoid deficiency — F

  They include disorders of glucocorticoid *excess*, e.g. Cushing's disease
- Phaeochromocytoma — T
- Primary hyperaldosteronism with excess mineralocorticoid secretion — T

Chapter 25

1 The main source of leptin is the hypothalamus — F

   The main source of leptin is adipose tissue

2   Leptin stimulates appetite   ☐F

   Leptin *depresses* appetite

3   Leptin's site of action for suppressing appetite is the hypothalamus   ☐T

4   Leptin downregulates hypothalamic endocannabinoid expression   ☐T

5   Leptin stimulates angiogenesis in endothelial cells   ☐T

A   Leptin inhibits the activity of neurones which express:

•   Neuropeptide Y   ☐T

•   Agouti-related peptide   ☐T

•   α-MSH   ☐F

   Leptin *increases* the activity of α-MSH-secreting neurones

B   Adiponectin:

•   Is a hormone secreted by adipose cells   ☐T

•   Decreases tissue sensitivity to insulin   ☐F

   Adiponectin *increases* tissue sensitivity to insulin, thus protecting against type 2 diabetes mellitus

•   Promotes triglyceride clearance   ☐T

•   Promotes glucose uptake into adipose tissue   ☐T

•   Suppresses glycogenolysis in liver   ☐T

•   Increases fatty acid uptake from blood into muscle   ☐T

•   Protects blood vessel endothelium from plaque formation   ☐T

C   High-risk factors associated with obesity include:

•   Hypotension   ☐F

   Hypertension is a high-risk factor with obesity

•   Breast cancer   ☐T

•   Coronary heart disease   ☐T

•   Type 2 diabetes mellitus and insulin resistance   ☐T

•   Heart failure   ☐T

•   Hypolipidaemia   ☐F

   Hyperlipidaemia is a high-risk factor with obesity

•   Kidney problems   ☐T

•   Baldness   ☐F

   Obesity is associated with *hirsutism* in women

•   Mobility problems   ☐T

•   Osteoarthritis   ☐T

•   Stroke   ☐T

D   Endocrine components of the 'metabolic syndrome' include:

•   Hypocortisolism   ☐F

   ***Hypercortisolism* is a component**

•   Glucose intolerance   ☐T

- Insulin resistance and hyperinsulinaemia   T
- Hypertriglyceridaemia   T
- Raised LDL and lowered HDL   T

Chapter 26

A The parathyroid glands:
- Are situated below the thyroid gland   F

  The parathyroids are embedded in the thyroid gland
- Secrete parathyroid hormone (PTH)   T

B Parathyroid hormone:
- Decreases Ca^{2+} concentrations in the blood   F

  PTH *increases* Ca^{2+} concentrations in the blood
- Decreases PO_4^{3-} concentrations in the blood   T
- Increases plasma Ca^{2+} by:
  - stimulating kidney production of vitamin D   T
  - mobilisation of Ca^{2+} from bone   T
  - enhancing tubular re-absorption of Ca^{2+} T

C PTH release:
- Is decreased by low extracellular Ca^{2+} concentrations   F

  PTH is *increased* by low extracellular Ca^{2+} concentrations
- Is partly controlled by a Ca^{2+} sensor receptor on the parathyroid cell   T

D PTH effects on bone:
- Are relatively slow   F

  PTH effects are relatively *fast* – release of Ca^{2+} from bone within minutes
- Include bone remodelling   T
- Result in bone resorption by osteoclasts   T

E The mechanism of action of PTH:
- Is through membrane-bound type I/type II PTH receptors   T
- Is also through:
  - type I PTH receptors are G-protein coupled and activate both cyclic AMP and IP_3 second messenger systems   T
  - type I PTH receptors are expressed poorly in bone   F

  Type I PTH receptors are expressed *mainly* in bone

F In primary hyperparathyroidism:
- Hypercalcaemia is caused by under-secretion of PTH   F

  There is *over*-secretion of PTH
- The cause is usually a malignant PTH-secreting adenoma   F

  It is usually a *benign* PTH-secreting adenoma among the parathyroid cells
- The disorder is more common in women   T

G Symptoms of primary hyperparathyroidism:
- Are similar to those of hypercalcaemia   `T`
- Include:
  - bone softening (osteomalacia)   `T`
  - osteoporosis   `T`
  - arthritis   `T`
  - osteitis fibrosa cystica (inflammation of bone)   `T`

H Effects of hypercalcaemia on the gastrointestinal tract include:
- Acute pancreatitis   `T`
- Diarrhoea   `F`
  Effects include *constipation*
- Nausea and vomiting   `T`
- Peptic ulceration   `T`

I Effects of hypercalcaemia on the central nervous system include:
- Ataxia, unsteady gait; difficulty with balance   `T`
- Hyperactivity   `F`
  Energy loss and fatigue occur
- Coma   `T`
- Delirium   `T`
- Depression   `T`
- Memory loss   `T`
- Psychosis (loss of contact with reality)   `T`

J Secondary hyperparathyroidism is usually secondary to renal failure,
   when the kidneys:
- Over-secrete active vitamin D   `F`
  The kidneys *fail to* secrete active vitamin D[1]
- Fail to secrete phosphate adequately[2]   `T`

K Tertiary hyperparathyroidism:
- May result from:
  - establishment of autonomous PTH gland activity disconnected
    from circulating PTH levels   `T`
  - resetting of the Ca^{2+} effect on bone   `T`
- Is possibly diagnosed on the basis of an inability to treat hypercalcaemia
  and osteomalacia with vitamin D therapy   `T`

---

[1] Active vitamin D suppresses expression of PTH by inhibiting transcription of PTH mRNA.

[2] Increased plasma phosphate promotes formation of insoluble calcium phosphate, thus removing Ca^{2+} from the circulation.

L Parathyroid-hormone-related protein (PTHrP):

- Is produced only by parathyroid cells   `F`

  PTHrP seems to made by virtually every tissue in the body

- Exists in several forms   `T`
- Binds to both the type I PTH and PTHrP receptors   `T`
- Has many actions, including:
  - control over cellular differentiation, proliferation and cell death   `T`
  - relaxing smooth muscle   `T`

M Refer to Figure 26.2, p. 184, for the correct labelling of this figure

Chapter 27

1 Calcitonin is synthesised in clear (C) cells in the thyroid gland   `T`
2 Calcitonin is a lipoprotein hormone   `F`

Calcitonin is a 32-amino acid polypeptide

3 Calcitonin is derived from a precursor called procalcitonin   `T`
4 Calcium acts through an intracellular receptor linked to the cyclic AMP system   `F`

It acts through an *extracellular* membrane-bound receptor

A Calcitonin's actions include:

- Reduction of blood calcium by:
  - increasing bone osteoclast activity   `F`

  Actions include *decreasing* bone osteoclast activity, thus protecting bone against demineralisation

  - reducing Ca^{2+} absorption from the GIT   `T`
  - reducing Ca^{2+} reabsorption from the kidney tubules   `T`
- Promotion of vitamin D production   `T`
- Possibly acting as a satiety hormone, reducing dietary Ca^{2+} intake `T`

B Uses of calcitonin (prescribed as salmon calcitonin) include:

- Treatment of bone metastases   `T`
- Treatment of postmenopausal osteoporosis   `T`
- Hypocalcaemia   `F`

  Uses include *hypercalcaemia*

- Protection against bone loss during illness and immobility   `T`

Chapter 28

1 Vitamin D is a collective term for different forms of calciferol   `T`
2 The active form of vitamin D is 1,25-dihydroxyvitamin D_3 `T`
3 1,25-dihydroxyvitamin D_3 is also called calcitriol   `T`

4　7-dehydrocholesterol conversion to vitamin D_3 is blocked by sunlight　☐F

　　The reaction is *stimulated* by sunlight

5　Cholecalciferol is converted to 25-hydroxycholecalciferol in the liver　☐T

6　25-hydroxycholecalciferol is converted to active vitamin D in the kidney, stimulated by parathyroid hormone (PTH)　☐T

7　Some food sources of vitamin D include milk, eggs, fish liver oils　☐T

8　Calcitonin is the major regulator of vitamin D production in the kidney　☐F

　　***PTH* is the major regulator of vitamin D production in the kidney**

9　Vitamin D acts through an intracellular cytoplasmic receptor　☐T

10　The receptor–vitamin D complex alters nuclear gene expression　☐T

A　Physiological actions of vitamin D include:

- Inhibition of calcium absorption from the GIT　☐F

  Actions include *promotion* of calcium absorption from the GIT

- Stimulation of calcium resorption from bone　☐T

- Stimulation of proteins mediating Ca^{2+} transport across gut membranes　☐T

- It may promote Ca^{2+} reabsorption in the kidneys　☐T

B　Causes of vitamin D deficiency include:

- Ageing　☐T

- Dietary deficiencies　☐T

- Chronic diseases e.g. cancer, diabetes, kidney damage　☐T

- Liver cirrhosis　☐T

- Mutations of the vitamin D receptor　☐T

- Rheumatoid arthritis　☐T

- Scanty clothing　☐F

  Causes of vitamin D deficiency include clothing that bars sunlight from most of the body

Chapter 29

1　An osteoblast is a cell that resorbs bone　☐F

　　An osteoblast produces and lays down bone; an *osteoclast* resorbs bone

2　Osteoporosis is the loss of bone causing fragile, brittle bones　☐T

3　Primary osteoporosis is considered to be caused by ageing　☐T

4　Secondary osteoporosis is caused by other health problems　☐T

5　Diagnosis of osteoporosis uses DEXA scans and through fractures from falls when standing　☐T

6　Paget's disease is a disorder of bone remodelling without reference to the body's requirements　☐T

7　Paget's disease occurs predominantly in women　☐F

　　Both sexes are equally at risk

A   Treatment of osteoporosis is mainly:
- Preventive with calcium and vitamin D supplements ⬜T
- HRT using synthetic estrogens or SERMs ⬜T
- Use of bisphosphonates, e.g. sodium alendronate ⬜T
- Teriparatide, an analogue of PTH ⬜T
- Calcitonin as a supplement to other treatments ⬜T
- Oral strontium ranelate ⬜T

B   Symptoms of osteoporosis may include:
- Loss of sensation in bone and joints ⬜F
  There is *pain* in bone and joints due to nerve compression
- Inflammation and swelling at joints ⬜T
- Abnormal skull shape ⬜T
- Heart problems ⬜T
- Fractures ⬜T

C   Paget's disease is diagnosed using:
- X-ray ⬜T
- Bone scans using radioactive isotopes e.g. gallium-67 ⬜T
- Blood levels of alkaline phosphatase, which is reduced in Paget's disease ⬜F
  Blood levels of alkaline phosphatase are *raised*

D   Paget's disease may be treated:
- With nothing if the patient is unaffected ⬜T
- For pain if needed ⬜T
- With bisphosphonates ⬜T
- Surgically if there is bone damage or deformity ⬜T

Chapter 30

1   An autosome is a sex chromosome ⬜F
     An autosome is any chromosome *other than* a sex chromosome
2   A neuroma is a tumour derived from a nerve cell ⬜T
3   MEN type 1 is also called Wermer's syndrome ⬜T
4   MEN type 1 affects the thyroid, pancreas and pituitary ⬜F
     MEN type I affects the *parathyroid*, pancreas and pituitary
5   MEN type 2 is also called the Sipple syndrome ⬜T
6   MEN type 2 is further subdivided into 2A and 2B ⬜T
7   MEN 2B is the most dangerous ⬜T

A   MEN 2A includes:
- Medullary thyroid cancer ⬜T
- Phaeochromocytoma ⬜T

- Parathyroid tumours, secreting calcitonin $\boxed{F}$

  MEN 2A includes parathyroid tumours, secreting *PTH*

B   MEN 2B includes:
- Phaeochromocytoma $\boxed{T}$
- Medullary thyroid cancer $\boxed{T}$
- Mucosal neuromas $\boxed{T}$
- Marfanoid features $\boxed{T}$

Index